DISMANTLING
the
Disability

MY UPHILL BATTLE WITH FRIEDREICH'S ATAXIA

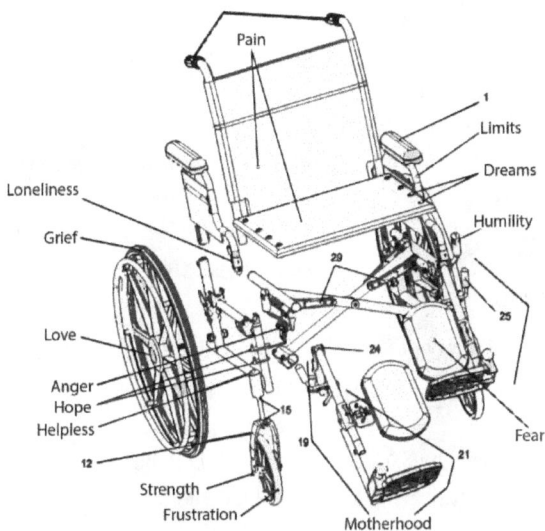

A MEMOIR BY
ERIN K. PIEPER

SMOKEBLOOD PUBLISHING
CASPER, WY

Smokeblood
Dismantling The Disability

Copyright ©2022 Erin K Pieper

All rights reserved.

This book is memoir. It reflects the author's present recollections of experiences over time. Some names and characteristics have been changed, some events have been compressed, and some dialogue has been recreated.

ISBN-13: 979-8-9851234-2-5

Library of Congress Control Number:
2021924475

Published by SMOKEBLOOD Publishing
Casper, WY | smokeblood.com

Exterior cover + interior cover page design by Colt McMurry
Cover design © Smokeblood, 2022
Edited by Marissa Waraksa

First Edition
Printed in the United States of America

ADVANCE PRAISE
FOR

Dismantling The Disability

"What a beautiful book. I was fully immersed within the first few pages. Erin's story is educational, witty, and poignant. She invites the reader into her life, sharing the trials, burdens, and beauty of it all. Erin has a gift with words, and I thank her for sharing them with the world. I highly recommend it!"
—Lisa M Brennan, author of *The Auditorium in My Mind: Treasuring My Transgender Child*

"This book is a beautiful and moving read! So graciously written, yet honest! Erin delivers a humbling perspective on life that one could benefit from striving to acquire."
—Rachael Cradic

"When living with Friedreich's Ataxia, it can feel like difficulty and darkness surround you—especially when you can no longer do simple things you could previously do. It can seem even darker if you are a parent. Erin's story serves as the light that shines through that darkness. We can't control how FA will affect us, but we can control our reaction to it. From my experience and from what Erin shows, a positive mindset and acceptance is key to navigating a life with Friedreich's Ataxia."
—Beverlee Blackston, diagnosed with FA

"Erin pours her heart and positivity into everyone she loves and everything she does. This book feels like a conversation with Erin; one you will be glad you showed up for. She pulls back the curtain on what it's like to live the *Mama Lifestyle*—changing diapers, making meals, driving to school and activities, and the like—all while battling a serious, degenerative disease. She shows up at six am every day and pushes herself to the limits to nurture and provide for her sweet and energetic son, and all from the discomfort of her wheelchair. Taking the time to read this book and experience the world through Erin's eyes will open your own. Diversity, equity, and inclusion have been in the spotlight recently, and rightly so; but time and again, the disabled are left out of advocacy circles. *Dismantling the Disability* is a moving story to take in and Erin's voice is a vital one to be heard."
—Katie Rengel

"Honest, thoughtful, and hopeful. *Dismantling the Disability* truly takes a deep dive into living life with a disability. Erin wonderfully and beautifully expresses her opinions and explores her feelings about Friedreich's Ataxia, being a mom, loneliness, togetherness, therapy, dating, participating in research, and so much more."

—Michael Gehr, diagnosed with FA

"Mothering is hard. Single mothering is even harder. Tack on a progressively degenerative disease crippling every aspect of your body's physical faculty, and you've got one hell of a daily grind. Despite inheriting a not-so-golden ticket, Erin Pieper relishes life and gracefully out-maneuvers her challenges with creativity, wit, and undying positivity. Whether you're looking for inspiration, relatability as a mother or are an individual battling your own handicap, Erin's narration of life experiences offers a genuine glimpse into the world of a *she*ro and the caliber of parent and *human* that I aspire to be."

—Elise Hyman

"This book details how one woman's fight against a very rare disease has helped her learn that she can move mountains. The author tells of a story filled with a multitude of emotion after learning that, at a young age, she has a disease that will change her entire world and potentially end her life way before her light has fully burned out. However, she learns that she has the fire and fight within her to not just be an individual with a disability, but a warrior with a mission to help fight for a cause that can hopefully one day save her life. This is a story of heartbreak, love, acceptance, and finding a power that is stronger than words and physical strength will ever be."

—Alicia Laird

"This book was both easy and hard for me to read: Easy because it is so well written with all of Erin's thoughts, feelings, fears, hopes and dreams, as well as love as a single parent, daughter, and friend. It was hard to read mostly because it opened me up to her daily struggles, fears, and society's naïveté towards making our world easier for our handicapped individuals to navigate.
This book is written from the heart and soul of a beautiful person, both inside and outside. Erin has inspired and touched so many people, and I know this book will touch the hearts of all who read her words. It was my honor to read her book, as she took me deeper into her world."

—Terie Pieper

DEDICATION

To my **son**, my love, my favorite Deputy—you're my constant source of inspiration. I will always strive for the stars for *you*.

And to my amazing **mom** who has stepped in to lend both helping hands so that I can grow and share my life, in hopes to make a positive impact.

CONTENTS

The world never stops moving.

Even if you feel you're frozen or pausing time for whatever reason, society keeps on living. It can be hard to jump back in. For this reason, I do my best to keep active in society. I don't want fear to overcome me or to see myself become this secluded person, anxious about life.

I know I push myself hard and believe humans can push themselves higher, faster—further than they give themselves credit for. The reason most don't push harder is fear. They come into new territory, and they don't know what the outcome will be, so they psych themselves out of it.

Like the famous quote of Erin Hanson goes:
"What if I fall? *Oh, but my darling, what if you fly?*"

—Erin K Pieper

FOREWORD

I've known Erin through every phase of her life: childhood, adulthood, motherhood. We have that special kind of friendship that works like muscle memory because it has been intact for so long.

When we were ten years old, Erin told me she wanted to have five kids by the time she was twenty. I remember panicking and saying, "What about college?" Even at the ripe age of ten, the expectations were real... and we quickly revised that number to twenty-five. Five kids and a husband by twenty-five. I had no such goals but remember vividly sitting in awe of how much family meant to Erin.

Twenty years have gone by, and Erin is the most resilient human and empathetic mother I know.

Her plan may not have worked out exactly as expected——thanks to Friedreich's Ataxia——but she has continued to live her life as a beautiful work in progress. Motherhood is hard without a life altering disability, yet Erin has faced and overcome so much to show up for her family. She doesn't take that job lightly and shares the struggles and victories of how resilience has guided her through early motherhood and led to an unbreakable bond with her son and family.

Anyone who knows Erin would describe her as inspirational and incredibly optimistic. She is all of those things, but this book reveals the struggle underneath the smile that she pushes through every day to overcome impossible odds and enjoy everything life has to offer. The vulnerability that Erin brings to her story is a true testament to how facing hard things has defined her life and brought her such power and resilience. This book is brave, and Erin's words are raw, revealing what it looks like to stare fear in the face and choose to live beyond it.

There were so many times over the years where Erin could have easily said, "I'm not up to come out tonight," or "I just can't do that;" but instead, she has chosen to navigate the complexities of life in a wheelchair as a challenge worth overcoming and celebrating. That is the power of choice, of resilience. The power of taking back the reins of life when given an impossible destiny.

In a world preoccupied with introspective worries and unaccomplished goals, Erin's perspective is a breath of fresh air. She gives us permission to accept ourselves wherever we're at, be authentic to what we need and live life having gratitude and empathy for others.

As a mother and FA advocate, Erin's mission is to destigmatize disability and that starts with education. This book takes an important look at the inside world of Friedreich's Ataxia. I encourage you to absorb it and share that knowledge.

Erin's story is a reminder that we are all capable of overcoming what seem to be insurmountable challenges. Whether you are living with a disability or are looking for some much-needed perspective, this book is a gentle guide on that journey—a lived experience that doesn't judge, but gently accepts circumstances for what they are to move forward.

Thank you, Erin, for sharing your wisdom with us in this powerful book. Enjoy!

Cheers,

Kat Earls

P.S. It's easy to get caught up in the perceived challenges of modern life, especially as a working mom. The endless ticker of to-do items that never get done, that email you didn't send, did you say that the right way in the meeting? If this book taught me anything, it's that these things do not matter. Appreciating your people, showing up always for those you love, and never giving up are what truly have an impact on your days here.

PREFACE

The Fall

I t's January of 2017. It's dark. It's cold. I pull into the driveway and have Eli with me in the car. We're getting out, and my mom comes out of the house to help get Sylvia for me from the back seat. I can do it on my own, but it's nice when someone is around to step in and help.

My mom gets Sylvia and brings her around to me, outside by the driver's seat. Eli is around four years old at the time, and able to walk into the house by himself, so in he goes while I get out. My mom walks beside me, as it's rather dark out, sort of guiding me and Sylvia towards the front door, around the bumps in the pavement.

As I move with Sylvia, she gets just a touch ahead of me, so my arms extend out to meet her. When I go to take the steps to catch up to where she is, I start to feel off balance and experience the sinking sensation of knowing that I am about to fall. When that sets in, I try to keep a swagger moving back and forth with Sylvia in a desperate attempt at counterbalance. I even lift her up as I feel myself shifting forwards, backwards, forwards, and backwards while I work to stabilize myself, but just *know* I am eventually going to fall, regardless.

There's always this thought that pops into your head when you know it's about to happen; like, *How do I wanna fall? On my bum? On my side? I obviously don't wanna fall face first or tense up.* You have this checklist go off in your head, because you know that if you go limp and just let it happen, your chances of getting hurt are quite slim. But if you try to catch yourself, and tense up; sure enough, something bad is bound to go down.

When I took that last teeter forward before the fall, I just braced myself, thinking, "This is it. It's gonna happen now."

When I grabbed Sylvia, I must have pulled her too close to my chest. I fell forwards over her as she jammed hard into my ribs and fell harder onto the pavement in front of me. As I fell forward, I jammed Sylvia even further in, and her cold, hard, aluminum bar just dug so deep into to my ribcage.

Sylvia is my walker.

As you may or may not know, there's a bar that runs across the top front of any walker. I fell forward hard over that thing, as the bar jammed itself into my ribcage and my body flipped over the bar and walker.

As I got closer to the ground, I let go of Sylvia and pulled my arms up and into my body in front of me. Thankfully, I caught myself with my arms, so I didn't face-plant onto the pavement, and instead landed on all fours. The bar of my walker was dug under one of my ribs as I landed there.

I started saying to my mom, "I think I broke a rib. I think I broke a rib." Over and over again, I said it.

I honestly think I was just saying it out of pure panic, at the time, because it was such a big fall. I was crying, and frustrated. It's a punch to the gut when I fall because it's this little reminder to me that I'm getting worse. *Why was I able to take that big of a step and get away with it yesterday, and the day before that, but not today?*

When I fall doing something I normally do, it's like, "*Shit*, I'm getting worse. I wasn't able to stabilize myself today like I could yesterday and the day before that and the day before that."

My mom said, "Alright, just gather yourself. Take your time, gather your thoughts and I'll help you up when you're ready." So I sat there crying hysterically, because I knew something bad had happened, but I also just think I was embarrassed. Even though it was only my mom, I felt embarrassed. I thought, *Shit. I'm having a hard time, and now, here, I fell.*

You just feel kinda butt hurt. Disappointed. Dare I say… ashamed.

Anyway, I got up with her help and she slowly walked me and Sylvia to the front door. When we get to the front door, there's a dual staircase that goes up and down to the other floors. At that time, I was just using Sylvia and didn't need alternative assistance yet, so whenever I got home or left, someone would come to help me navigate the stairs.

My mom carried Sylvia upstairs while I held onto the railing and banisters to pull myself up the stairs on my own. But it hurt. It hurt *bad.* I could feel, with every step I took, that my ribs were super sore. So sore my body tensed in response with every micromovement I made.

When I got all the way up the stairs, I sat on the couch to start feeling around for what hurt. I knew intuitively that I had hurt myself but was trying to talk myself down from the idea of a broken rib. *Maybe I just bruised it. I probably did… but it does hurt bad.* So I pretty much just hung around on the couch for a few hours, resting and processing what had happened, and what could be wrong.

I was cut up with some blood on my hands, especially where my thumbs and my palm come together. It later bruised up there. I didn't hurt my knees; most of the pressure of the fall went into my hands and with my ribcage into Sylvia. It was the ribs I was really worried about.

I put some ice on my ribs, and days went by as I continued to convince myself that nothing was broken in the fall. But the pain was actually getting worse, so every time I inhaled or went to talk, it would just hurt so much. I'd get up and walk to use the bathroom, but wherever I went, I felt that sore, achy throb ripple across my torso.

A week after the fall, Eli was playing indoor soccer. Joey, his dad, decided to go with me to watch. The indoor facility had stairs, but no ramp or working elevator—nothing. He would usually carry me up the stairs, sort of tossing me over his shoulder, but this time around, my ribs were cutting into his shoulder the entire time. It hurt so, *so* much. He brought my wheelchair up the stairs afterwards for me to sit on, but I was still in extreme pain and discomfort.

The next few days, it only got worse. Pretty much everything I did started to come with a searing pain. I just couldn't get comfortable. When I moved, it hurt. When I slept, it hurt. When I breathed, or ate, or talked: it hurt. Everything.

After doing some self-research, I learned that the only way to heal a rib is to let it heal on its own. You can obviously take some pain meds or muscle relaxers for the pain, but that's pretty much it. So I decided to go into urgent care, hoping to come out of the visit with pain meds or something of the sort. I also wanted confirmation one way or the other, and hoped they would do an x-ray to determine whether a rib was broken or not.

And sure enough, you could see on the x-ray that one of my ribs had indeed chipped in the fall. The doctor said, "Time will heal," and prescribed me some muscle relaxers. But I didn't really like the drugs. I took a few for a couple of days, but when I took them, they did the opposite of what they were meant for. I was wide awake, anxious, and it wasn't calming me down or soothing my pain by any means.

What bugs me to think about is how, as the doctor informed me, the chipped-off piece of my rib bone was just floating around in my body now. They said it was no big deal, and that somehow the bone breaks down and you get rid of it. I don't remember how this works, or what this means. I imagine an animation of a piece of bone disintegrating or getting small enough to where you poop it out. I don't know, but I know I don't like it.

The doctor told me to ensure I didn't do any more harm to my injury, which turned out to be the hardest part since, when I use my walker, I use the force of my arms, which I could really feel into my ribcage in the weeks after the fall. Just getting up came with a searing pain, so I started to use the wheelchair more, taking more advantage of it. And as my rib started healing, I was still hesitant to do too much, or get up and walk, as I was obviously afraid that it could happen again. The pain was so intense, I never wanted to feel that again.

With the fall, I don't think my footing was off, or that my ankle rolled, or that my shoelace was untied and I had tripped on it. I don't think it was any of that. I think it was just feeling like I was in a hurry, and I probably was, knowing it was January, and it was cold, and it was winter.

I hate the winter so much, and when I'm cold it is actually harder for me to move because all of my muscles tense up. I'm sure that my mentality at the time was, *Let's get out of this car and get in the house as quickly as possible.* Hence why I was probably taking a bit too big of strides with Sylvia and too big of steps forward to meet her.

I was not being very careful or patient with myself. And with my condition, I always have to be careful and patient with myself.

When I take too big of strides like that, I have to concentrate a lot on making sure it's a sort of smooth glide, and I'm assuming that I was pretty jagged with my navigation at the time. And I was picking Sylvia up over the bumps, which I'm sure didn't help my balance it at all.

What I have found to be true is that when you're not as mobile as you once were, and you have a disease like I do, it will be harder to get back to where you were before a setback like this. That's why they always say to walk for as long as you can with a degenerative disease, because when you stop using the muscles that help, it's very difficult to get back to where you were—if you even *can* get it back.

In my case, I don't think I ever fully got back to where I was before the fall. Yeah, I'll get up here and there, like when I'm at the gym or getting out of the wheelchair to use the bathroom, or when I'm transitioning out of the wheelchair into the shower or when walking short distances. Stuff like that, but I never really went back to how I was, actively walking with Sylvia.

Just another loss I've had to bear, living with Friedreich's Ataxia.

I take the memory of my fall as a reminder that I need to get out of the wheelchair as often as I can, whether to stretch or move, or do whatever I can to get my legs moving and my heart pumping. Much like the saying, "If you don't use it, you lose it." I think that speaks volumes about someone who struggles with FA.

CHAPTER ONE

Is It Me, or Is It My Disease?

I am beyond grateful for my life. Grateful for what I *do* have, for all that I've overcome, and to simply be alive every day. Sometimes, I wonder if my disease is what has brought me into this place where I can choose gratitude over victimizing myself for all the challenges I've had to face. But one thing I'm still searching for solace within is whether some of the ways people treat me or engage with me have to do more with me, my personality, and my true self; versus how much of their behaviors are directly in response to my illness and all that exists in my life as a direct result.

How many times have relationships faltered, men simply drifting away from my life without any explanation or further contact? How many times have I felt that discomfort on the other line when I hear excuses why someone doesn't want to meet me, hang out, or why a group of friends has gotten together but didn't invite me? I wonder in my mind, *Is it because I come with a hassle?*

Is it just us drifting apart, or is it my disease pushing them away?

I don't want to make it all about my disease; maybe it's some other reason entirely. But the first thing I think of when these things happen is that it's because of my condition. It could be that I don't like their same kind of music, or conversation, or something just as remedial... but for me, it feels like, *Who'd want to deal with this if they didn't have to?*

I understand and accept their decisions either way; everyone is free to do what they like with their own relationships and lives, of course. But for my own reasons, I wonder. I wonder what in my life could be easier, better, or different... without my disease.

And I might as well get into it, right? My disease is called Friedreich's Ataxia, or FA for short (because, well, of course, who wants to pronounce all that). This disease, which has spanned the greater part of my life, time, and energy, comes with many debilitating symptoms.

I have to use a wheelchair to get around. I need assistance to do many basic, human tasks. I go to therapy to keep up with my body's evolving needs, and it takes me much longer to accomplish that which able-bodied people can do without a second thought. On top of it all, then there's other people's experiences with me as a disabled person. Navigating the world outside, with its many stairs, fast-paced people, and standard operating procedures that someone like me is just not designed to fit into.

I stand out, as most disabled individuals do. I simply cannot blend in, and I'm noticed as I move through my day-to-day life. But generally, it isn't for reasons I want to be noticed. More often than not, it's because I need *extra* [help, time, patience, you name it!]. So despite already having to deal with whatever symptoms accompany a condition; there's this stigma, socially, that disabled people must swim upstream against. I often feel… what's the best word… *unwanted* in society. I feel like a burden, on the whole.

I feel like—only sometimes—an inconvenience. I do my best to handle my own shit, but I do feel that people have to do "extra" for me, just for us to hang out and catch up. Whether they mind or not, sometimes it really hits me just how much I rely on someone wheeling me over their front porch step. This thought begs me to question, then, my self-worth and value. What could *I* offer to others in return?

I didn't do anything wrong to "deserve" this disease. I didn't ask for this. It just is. And as a result, yes, my life requires a lot of extra focus, a commitment to moving at my own pace (patience, patience, patience), and different expectations for myself and my life than an able-bodied person would traditionally possess.

I don't always feel as included as I would like. *Do they not want to have to help me? Would they rather enjoy being around the other able-bodied people instead, so they can just live their lives more comfortably? Do the guys I date feel like they would rather lock arms with someone walking in the park than have to wheel someone around all their life?*

These questions don't fill my days or flood my thoughts too often. I am, quite honestly, both proud and grateful for the life I lead. But sometimes, when my challenges get the best of me, I'm by myself facing a newly tedious task, or I simply feel overwhelmed, it's hard *not* to compare myself to my own memory and the social reminders of what it's like to be an able-bodied person moving through the world today. It's difficult not to wonder or contemplate the space between.

In the now, I am grateful for the incredible friendships and close emotional bonds I've been able to have in my life. Encouragement from loved ones has kept me strong, helped me build up resilience as I need it, and has even motivated me to write this book.

Years ago, I started a personal blog (mywobblyworld.com), and it became a hobby I turned out to be pretty damn good at. I wanted to educate as many people as I could about the rarity of the disease I'd inherited, as well as share my stories of juggling single motherhood through it all.

I like to have a sense of humor while expressing my thoughts and feelings in as relatable and raw of a way as I can, and I've found that writing about the realness of FA and parenthood has allowed me the space to do just that! As more posts were written on the blog, I generated a small fan base, met wonderful other individuals with FA, answered many curiosities about having children in my condition and, quite importantly, educated and spread awareness about a disease most know nothing about.

With the impact of many months of quarantine and only my son's virtual schooling to focus on, I finally took all the encouragement from my blog and decided to pour more knowledge and love into something bigger: this book! I began my hunt for an editor, proofreader, publisher—just any professional guidance I needed to formulate a complete book—and began the process of writing down literally anything that popped into my head.

I spent enormous amounts of time typing in the Notes app on my phone because, with my disease, using my thumbs to type is quicker and more coordinated than using a computer. As I'll unveil throughout the book, FA causes coordination to deteriorate, so using my phone to get my words out was a blessing. Plus, it gave me the liberty to add to a chapter whenever I had a thought while driving, and could simply pull over to type away.

Writing a book is probably one of the most challenging, but rewarding experiences I've taken on, and I am very thankful to myself for being patient and expanding my creative awareness in this way. There were, of course, days where I couldn't even think about writing and wanted to give up and throw my phone or computer out the window—whether due to self-doubt or my own life overwhelm—but I am so happy that I kept pushing forward. Mostly for you, so you could have this fabulous book to read (at least, I think it's fabulous) and so that I could inform any and all potential readers about this lesser-known illness and what it's like to live through my body. I also want to show other individuals with FA—and the whole world for that matter—that you can, in fact, have children, even if you have FA or a disability like mine; even if you raise them as a single parent.

I truly dedicate my perseverance and ability to communicate deeply about FA to my son. I want him to feel like his Mama did great things in this world and used her voice to enlighten others to feel less awkward and uncomfortable around disabilities.

My writings, whether in the blog or this book, will shed much light on my life pre-FA and pre-baby, up until present day. How I've handled my diagnosis; how having a child was and still is tough. I hope reading this will enlighten your thought process on disabilities or give you a sense of relatability to debilitating diseases, or else answer your "What if's"—or all the above!

My *reason* for sharing this book is to stop hiding behind closed doors and stop feeling so alone with this disease and the dynamics I face. The only way anyone can relate to or understand something is if someone speaks up about it. I know, over the years, I've shed some knowledge and positivity through my blog, as well as my involvement in particular organizations and groups; now I feel I can reach even more people and raise my platform with this book. I wish to uplift and give a platform to the voices of FA.

Not everyone faced with FA can or will be able to speak out or be a leader of some sort, so I feel I've been given a strong voice for a reason. The reason I'm concluding to is enlightening as many people as I can on this disease, all while bringing a voice to the potentially voiceless. Plus, my dynamic becomes all the more touching as it comes to light how I am going through this physical disability while being a single mom.

Disabilities definitely do not have to define you, but just because I come off as a fighter, I still battle with the overbearing thoughts… that FA wins at times. I don't know if that will 100%

ever go away, but how I deal with the thoughts and act upon them is what matters. My attitude is probably one of my strongest attributes in how it allows me to face and navigate my illness, time and time again. I am reminded, literally every second, of FA: All my body's movements are the way they are because of FA.

I deeply enjoy my alone time. I am not a secluded person, nor do I hide out from society; I just really enjoy *me time*, you know? When I'd started my blog in 2015, I received a lot of recognition in support of my writing a book; when, during the Covid-19 pandemic, I really missed that alone time, I realized it was perfect timing for me to finally start writing. I felt that it would be a big release for me to write everything out—while my son was virtually learning nearby. It was like we were both doing our homework together. I kinda loved it!

It was hard to concentrate sometimes, hearing him talk to his class, so I'd do my best and practice tuning him out to focus on the writing. Those times where I wanted to give up, my kiddo kept me going. I know it's cliche, but my son has been the reason for so much of my motivation. Parents are the best role models for their kids, and it will be wonderful for him to see how much effort I put into making a positive difference in the world.

My story is most unique because of my child. Not many people correlate a physical disability with having kids. Disabilities are generally accompanied by a quick judgment of sadness, and seeing one as being dependent and not fitting into society. But the more it's talked about, the less awkward people will feel as their mind shifts to a better understanding, being more open-minded around disabilities.

I want as many people to be educated on disabilities as they are in basic math. How awesome would it be to have classes in elementary, middle, and high schools teaching as much as possible about understanding disabilities?! Not only in college when you're studying to be a counselor or social worker or doctor… but for everyone! A standard of awareness across the board. Learning about things when you're young sets a pattern of behavior and perspective that is carried through the rest of your life, and I feel we really need—that it's truly time—to shift the paradigm.

When I'm with my son Eli, around his friends or at his school, I know I probably have surprised, and perhaps influenced youngsters' emotions when they see me in a wheelchair. They've probably not seen the mom of a young child in a wheelchair before; while Eli, on the other end, is learning how to be more understanding and help push me up a hill, open the door wider for me or reach for something I cannot. I would think it would open their minds toward capabilities overall so that they understand it more deeply as they grow. I feel that even my presence may plant the seed for change in their lives.

So in this book, I'll share my story. My life story, which just so happens to have been seriously influenced by the symptoms of my disease. *My* FA. It's mine. It is entwined within me, sometimes blurring the distinctions between myself and my disease.

Am I my disease? Yes and no. From one perspective, I am. From another, I am not. I toggle between the two, and am still searching for clarity through it all.

This book is part memoir, part informant; part question, part answer. I've learned a lot about myself and my disease through the journey I share in the following chapters. Overall, my mission with this book is to break the stigmas, question the status quos of my disease, and all diseases, and unpack some of the complexities I've come up against.

I hope for you to find what you're looking for; the answer to the question that led you to pick up this book in the first place. I hope for you to learn a thing or two that's new, and I hope that you come to find clarity around disabilities and capabilities by the time you flip the final page. Thank you for reading, thank you for caring, and *thank you* for showing up here. Enjoy!

CHAPTER TWO

The Start of Life

E very life has a beginning. Mine started five days before Christmas in the late '80s in St. Louis, Missouri. My uncle was the very first person to see me take my first breath in this big world. As weird as that may sound, he was a great OBGYN with no blood relation to my mom: Dr. S., known as Uncle Mario to me, is married to my dad's sister.

I was *literally* born to family—by which, I mean the hands who delivered me were family—and thus, I live by the importance of the slogan: 'Family Is Everything.' I learned from quite a young age to keep family close and always support them in whatever way possible.

I am the first and last child born to my parents, Kirk and Pam. They were each married previously, and each has a son with their exes, so I have two older half-brothers, Peter and Ryan. Peter comes from my mom and Ryan, my dad.

Peter lived with us before becoming an adult, so he's the one I remember most. He's nine-and-a-half years older than me. Through my youth, he was off enjoying his teen years, in and out of the room down the hall, until he started his new journey at eighteen in California. With the age gap, we obviously were at different levels with our passions, but he was very caring and attentive to me, especially so while I was young. Ryan, about eight years my senior as well, never lived close by. Though he and I have spent more time connecting on our lives and sharing pictures of our kids as of late, Ryan lived down in Florida with his mom while we were young. So I basically grew up as an "only child" in my home.

However, I was surely not exposed to that level of isolation. I always had access to quite a large family on my dad's side, as my dad is one of eight siblings, and we would get together with most

21 | P a g e

of them and their families often. I have, thus, also been fortunate to have multiple handfuls of cousins—many around my age. Growing up and to this day, we still show love, support, and enjoy each other's company.

With my dad's side of the family being so large, there was hardly a birthday, Thanksgiving, Christmas, or Easter not celebrated. Even random get-togethers happened often, such as dinners, sporting events, trivia nights, school functions, baptisms, graduations, showers, weddings, funerals… you name it, I'm sure some of the family, if not most, were celebrating it all together.

If my mom's family had lived nearby, we'd have had that same pep to see them often, too. To this day, my mom has a brother and some cousins who live in her home state of Connecticut. When her parents and extended family were living, they had resided in Connecticut also. She's the one that got away! We—although mostly mom—have keep in contact the best we can through phone calls, gifts in the mail, and trips to visit one another whenever possible, but I know she still yearns to see them more.

My parents met in Miami, FL, where they'd both lived in the early '80s. They each had recently divorced their first spouses, and I would imagine, were giving the cat-and-mouse flirtation a rather cute look. My mom and Peter went to a restaurant on Mother's Day to celebrate, and Kirk just so happened to be their waiter. He gave my mom a rose—as that was what the restaurant gave to all mothers who were dining that day—but from what I've gathered, the gesture brought on some initial sparks. From then on, Pam and Peter became regulars, always requesting to sit in Kirk's section. The romance blossomed, they dated, fell in love, all three of them moved to my dad's hometown, mom became pregnant with me, they got married, and the rest is *my* story to tell!

Now, who *am* I? This author you've come to read about; the woman with a story important enough to describe in detail in a book? Before we get into the meat of it all, I bet it would be nice to see some context of where I'm coming from; of who I even am! But you know, this is one of the toughest ideas I've considered since beginning to write my memoir. This ever-elusive question, though, does come with the task of constructing any memoir: "How would you describe yourself?"

Why is it that I stutter, sweat, and bounce around that question so much? It should be simple, yet it's so damn difficult for me to answer. To come up with the clarity of how I would choose to define myself.

I would say I am a fun-loving, high-spirited, sociable, glass-half-full kind of gal. I have strong beliefs and opinions, but always leave room for someone to bring other points of view to the table. I'll put in hard work, even if I hate it. I'm loyal and do my darndest to do what I say I will, and live through my actions, and not just my words. I have manners—a huge thing in my book—am extremely empathetic and shed a tear even at the sight of anyone hurt or lost in their own suffering.

I have zero tolerance for bullies, especially when it's happening to kids at school! I try not to complain about anything, but sometimes I've just gotta let it out, vent, and release the pressure. [Sorry—not sorry!] I can see the merit of both political parties. Each offers some good, solid points I can support, while each also includes some things I can't support. I believe in God. I am a Christian and know the ways prayer can be powerful. Science is awesome and cool, but not always the right or only answer. Love is Love—all deserve happiness. Black Lives Matter, but so do Blue (law enforcement, if you're unfamiliar with the phrase).

I have a large family, and so some are die-hard liberals while others are quite conservative. I tend to stay in the middle of the road and always keep an open mind with politics, especially when my family members discuss their perspectives of choice. I hate seeing the family argue and put each other down because of their political beliefs—maybe that's why I can't pick a side—because my family is either far left or far right and it irks me to see them get so caught up in the debates. I prefer "pro-life," but have no judgment if you're "pro-choice." It's a complex issue, and truly it's your body to choose with, not mine. Color, religion, ethnicity, and sexuality hold no difference in my book. Be you. Be your absolutely, totally unique self and choose to be wholly proud of yourself for it!

If anything, that's my *stance*: You be you, and be confident in that!

I'm somebody who likes the warmth and spending time outside. I really do believe I'm a very open and relaxed person. I can find enjoyment in just about everything. I enjoy alone time, small crowds, large crowds, one-on-one time—you name it, I really can go with the flow and enjoy the company of whoever's around me. I'm someone who enjoys a good wine paired with a TV series to binge on, and just as much, to spontaneously go out with friends or laugh with my son at the newest TikTok challenges.

I absolutely love talking with Eli. My favorite memories are of us lying in bed, cuddled under the blankets with our pillows perfectly touching, corner-to-corner, while we talk about whatever's on his mind. He always wants me to tell him a "bedtime story" about something I went through at a particular age. He may say, "Tell me a story from when you were fifteen...." I love sharing my life stories with him.

I'm sure Eli knows every detail about my life by now and it surely is one of my favorite bonds that we share. I love how deep and honest he can be, and how he trusts me wholeheartedly. I always reassure him that I won't tell anyone about what he shares. I'm sure the older he gets, the more boundaries and rules will be set to limit this time—that is, if he still wants to chat with me the same way then!

But anyway, back to me. *See?!* I get so sidetracked. So: describing me... I absolutely love someone who takes charge. I'm always having to find the most accessible places and things, and it becomes monotonous and exhaustive after a while. I call and do the research necessary, but I really love feeling like I don't need to be on alert or in charge all of the time.

And I enjoy not taking things too seriously. Having more fun. Waking up naturally—no alarms necessary. Staying up past bedtime. I think I was meant to be a 60's baby, to be honest: The hippie van. No cell phones. No internet. "Fly by the seat of your pants" aligns as my motto, for sure. Be free. Throw up peace signs. In truth, I feel this is why I struggle so much with being disabled. Limited. Having to be so careful and aware so much of the time.

I like to just follow my intuition. And it usually doesn't steer me wrong! I live for the summers, and I absolutely love hearing the birds chirp and the hum of crickets at night. My favorite smell is vanilla. It's my mom's favorite scent and she loves burning vanilla candles—I always think of her when I smell it and she's one of my favorite humans, so of course I would love what she loves!

Another smell I really enjoy, oddly enough, is bacon. I don't eat meat anymore and could vomit thinking of putting red meat or chicken in my mouth, but the smell of bacon brings me to a warm and cozy place. Sundays in my family were and still are the offerings of the big-style breakfast: Eggs. Bacon. Toast. Hash browns. Freshly brewed coffee. It's the smell of family and I absolutely love my mom's tradition of Sunday breakfast, even though I just settle for cereal with banana nowadays. In fact, this is probably why breakfast food was my favorite while I was pregnant—it gave me a sense of security and family meaning.

My favorite sights are seeing my son do something he loves or being a wonderful friend. My heart is so happy, seeing my kid happy. My other favorite thing to see is palm trees. There's this feeling that overcomes me that everything is alright. I find myself really feeling the Bob Marley song *Every Little Thing is Gonna be Alright*.

Ever since my first trip to Florida, I fell in love with the "no shoes, no shirt, no problems" philosophy. I went to Florida often with my friend and her family when I was younger, and boy could we lie on the beach or park by the pool all day long, the both of us loving every minute of it. It wasn't uncommon for us to make friends with kids or teens our age who were vacationing at the same place as us, all becoming buddies for the week. We were the *cute girls*, so we got lots of attention and we ate it up while we could!

We were always the ones who could start a fun hangout on the beach after dark and find a way to sneak a few sips of alcohol. We were the fun, slightly bending the rules kind of chicks. Kat was and still is my best friend. Many of my favorite and most laughable moments have been with her. One night, when we were around seventeen, she let me pierce her belly button. All we had was a long sewing needle. She put lots of ice on her belly button to numb it, and then I jammed that needle through. The problem was—once I wiggled that needle through, I couldn't get the belly ring thru the hole, so we just left the needle in for the night. We ended up just taking it out the next day, so all that work was for nothing! Save for the epic memory, which tickles me every time I remember it.

We also went to Girl Scouts camp together where one night, Kat thought she could bungee jump off our cabin window and down to the woods, so she tied one of those bungee cords to the drawstring of her Umbro shorts and took the leap. They ripped from the crotch to the back, and she landed face-first on the ground. Nothing was hurt but her ego. Sometimes, when I need a good laugh, I return to that memory. It's one of those memories where I laugh so hard that I start to cry! Probably one of my top funniest moments ever.

When I was a kid and was asked the age-old question, "What do you want to be when you grow up?" I instantly could list off goals of my very own, and I had this yearning to do big things. I dreamt of being a mom of four or five kids, having a big career as a veterinarian, and finding a Prince Charming who would sweep me off my feet. And we'd live happily ever after in a mansion with multiple cars—at least that's what the childhood game M.A.S.H. taught me.

In my younger days I was shy, quiet, and a big worrywart. I was probably the most obedient little girl ever. My mom used to say how I would be the only kid in daycare who would clean up; the other kids wouldn't help, so I cleaned it all without a complaint. That was the kind of kid I was—always following the rules... at least until I became a teenager. I was and still am a mommy's girl, though. My mom's been my bestie since day one. I was definitely a girly girl, as well. I wasn't much for getting dirty or muddy; I enjoyed playing comfortably with my Barbie dolls for hours under the dining room table. I would just get lost in my own world forever, losing time, making play.

Fast forward to my teens: I went to an all-girls private catholic high school. It surely didn't mean I was a "goody-two-shoes" or "stuck up," in case that's your initial thought. My dad and his siblings were raised Catholic—as you can see in how my grandparents had eight children—and my mom was raised Catholic, as well, so they guided me to follow that same path. Being in St. Louis, that was very much the norm, anyways.

"Where did you go to high school?" is another norm and a common ice breaker across all of St. Louis. To answer it: I went to Notre Dame High School. There are tons of private Catholic schools here, and even elementary and middle schools, though most of us call it all "grade school." Mine was called Assumption. It was co-ed. The girls wore the classic plaid green jumpers or skirts with a white collared shirt, and the boys, blue slacks with the same white collared shirt. It wasn't much for fashion, but at least we didn't have to worry about picking out a new outfit every day.

I still possess the morals and manners that I credit to my schooling. "Please," "Thank You," eye contact, and "Excuse Me" go a long way, in my book. Addressing elders and friends' parents by "Mr., Mrs. or Ms." still stands for me, to this day. If I'd known you as an adult when I was younger, I probably still won't refer to you on a first-name basis.

Notre Dame, like many other Catholic High Schools in St. Louis, did not have tons of students. I would say maybe 400 girls in the whole place. I knew most of the girls' names but definitely recognized all the faces. I enjoyed going to an all-girls school; maybe it had more drama lurking in the halls, but without all the boy distractions to worry about. High School opened a whole new world for me. I literally came out of the woodworks right at the end of eighth grade: braces off, contacts in, tamed hair, and womanly body parts quite on point. I turned into a hottie pretty much overnight, and I didn't know at all how to handle it.

When I sprouted into my womanhood, my braces were removed to reveal a smile that started to draw people towards me. I noticed a definitive shift, though I do think the complement of my, as some have said, *piercing* blue eyes may have helped, now that there weren't any glasses blocking them from view.

My hair is brown by nature, but I had gotten caramel and blonde highlights as I turned this corner from girl into maiden, and it definitely added to the look, as it was really thick, long and lush. I had such a nice body and small frame, with about 110 pounds to me and a flat stomach I still dream about. All this and my arms, toned like a yogi, really started turning the attention of the guys.

I was a trend setter and probably a leader-type but humble about it because I don't feed off of that attention. Never have. But it is nice to be so well liked. Fitting in so well. Being looked at with affirmation and affection. I miss that now. Even though I still don't think I'm lacking in the beauty department, by any regard, I also think that my wheelchair gets between the guys and that piercing, blue-eyed smile I still possess.

I was a little rebellious back then, but never out of control or anything. I wanted my nose pierced when I was seventeen, but my parents didn't want me to. So of course, on my eighteenth birthday, I got it pierced without telling them. Even though I was legally an adult, I was nervous about their reaction. I wouldn't say they loved it, but they definitely learned to let it go and accept it.

I did smoke cigarettes for around five years but never could smoke in front of my parents or family. Not that they asked me not to; just out of respect, I couldn't do it or ever bluntly admit that I smoked. I am sure my parents knew because of the smell on me and the random burn holes I had on my seat in the car, but I never said to them, "I smoke." Luckily, I quit on my 23rd birthday. I had strep throat a week prior to my birthday and didn't smoke as I was recovering, even when I went out for my birthday with friends and partied at the bar. If you've ever smoked before, you may relate to wanting to light up once you've been drinking. I put myself to the test to see if I could refrain from smoking as I drank and I did! I told myself, *If I can do that, then I can keep trucking towards quitting.* I'm so happy I quit that habit. And sure, I'll have a cig here and there, but the need for it is completely gone.

I would sneak out of the house or sneak people in back then, too. And I've had plenty of fake IDs over the years, as well. One when I was sixteen or seventeen that said I was eighteen, just so I could buy cigarettes, and a couple when I was eighteen to twenty years old, to say I was twenty-one so that I could buy booze.

My IDs were golden because they were real and legit without scratch marks. I was able to find someone that resembled my look, height and weight so it passed 99% of the time. But there was one time where my ID didn't quite cut it because the gas station clerk recognized and knew the real person on my ID. She called me out, but before she could do anything else, I just grabbed the ID and walked out, and didn't go back there again.

By the time I turned twenty-one, the excitement to drink, be served, or buy it at a store wasn't too thrilling anymore. The moral standpoint felt good, that I was doing it truthfully and legally, but I partied so much starting at seventeen, so it was like, "Okay, I'm twenty-one now. No biggie."

I have a pretty laid-back personality. I love cracking jokes and am generally a fun person, so it was difficult for me to understand what a guy saw when he looked at me back then. I didn't know if it was just the looks they wanted, or whether it was my personality that really drew them toward me—or was it the whole package they desired? Beauty? Brains? Sass? To be honest, I wasn't extra smart. I was average in academics, so I'm not too sure they were blown away with that. Looking back, I wish I'd had more of a sense of when a guy was just being a jerk and only liked me for the way I looked.

Notre Dame has this fun fundraiser they put on every year called the Fall Festival. Each grade would have six cheerleaders, a "fall festival favorite" and two runners-up that the class would vote for, at least back in my day. Each grade would compete to raise the most money, and whoever won, their 'Favorite' would be crowned Queen. It was typically the Senior Class who won, and rightfully so. It was a good, clean competition that encouraged extreme school spirit to raise funds for Notre Dame. My freshman year, I tried out as a cheerleader and was chosen as one of the six. It was so much fun! We had to make up our cheers, team name, and design as well as make our own outfits. That's about as athletic as I was in high school, though. I played soccer and volleyball in grade school, but once I hit puberty, it was goodbye sports and hello makeup!

As my four wonderful years of High School came to an end, it was time to prepare for college.

I decided to go to college at Missouri State University (MSU) in Springfield, MO. Freshman year was one of the best years of my life. It was like I had discovered a whole new me. I lived in the dorms with a good friend from high school—the recipe for non-stop fun. I partied way too much and ended up missing a lot of classes. Skipping class quickly became a habit, and I started missing exams, or else would just totally guess at every answer, which generally awarded me a big, fat F. By the end of the semester, I ended up having a G.P.A. of 1.8. Quite embarrassing, I know. After finding out, I really wasn't prepared for what was to come; at that point, I was sure I would get kicked out.

And sure enough, after that semester ended, the Dean called me into his office and asked about my G.P.A. I was smart enough to convince him to give me a second chance, and he did. But he told me I was to maintain a G.P.A. of 2.5 or above for the rest of this, as well as the next, semester. It sounded like a fair deal to me, so we shook on it, and I held up my end of the bargain.

Things became more adventurous as I moved through college, and soon I started dating someone. He was someone to keep me grounded and motivated in keeping my grades up, so I didn't get the boot out of MSU. A year ahead of me, he helped me out with my projects and assignments from time to time. He was also part of a fraternity, so my party side still got to come out to play. I kind of had the best of both worlds—keeping my studies up while having the frat boys throw some pretty epic parties. I've always said that it's best to both work hard *and* play hard! That semester was definitely one of my favorite memories. I was able to maintain my G.P.A., learned to balance school and social life, and was over the moon in love with my boyfriend. I was only nineteen, but I thought I had it all together. Of course, I didn't—naïve for sure! All because I was on a high with my boyfriend, I was doing better in school, and just all around doing great. So here I thought I had all of the world's problems figured out and that life was pretty much perfect.

I think I was just so flipping happy. I felt like I *had it all*. I don't think I have had many times in my life when the world just seemed so easy, where I was over the moon happy. Of course, I feel that way about my son, but there are always hardships around me now, even though I have such unconditional love for my kid lighting up my life.

I would've loved to have frozen time for a bit and just stayed that content for a while. That blissfully satisfied. That whole. I call myself naïve, now, because I truly didn't believe that bad things would ever happen to me. But, oh boy, they would. Again and again, with momentum, it seemed, in the years to come.

At the end of the school year in May, my friend and I went back to St. Louis to live with our parents—my boyfriend stayed with his parents, further west; about 30 minutes from my parents—and I resumed work at a tanning salon I'd used to work at consistently before college. I'd started working there at sixteen, often left all alone to run the place by myself. Though it wasn't necessarily hard work, being the only one working during a shift definitely required me to "run" the salon. With so much authority, I just might have given a few extra friends-and-family discounts away—*Whoops!*

In short, it felt like I was taking charge of my life efficiently, even as I navigated life back in my hometown. And even though summer break was quite the slurry of emotions, as my boyfriend and I were in the midst of an "on-again-off-again" relationship.

The following semester, I began to have more, and newer responsibilities. I moved in with my dear friend Kristian from High School and one other friend we had made a year prior into a cute and newly built home about twenty minutes away from campus.

This newly found freedom and responsibility truly hit me. Now I was supposed to pay rent and buy groceries... all by myself. Not only that, but I had to pay to fill my gas tank regularly and pay all these bills. I realized, in order to pay for all of my expenses, I would have to work two jobs. During that time, I ended up juggling work and college. It became hard to find time between the two, and the final "off" with my boyfriend was the icing on that shitty, busy, overwhelming cake. The stress and heartbreak led to trips home to St. Louis for any weekend when I could get off from work.

I would just curl up in my bed and cry at this point. My world already felt like it was crumbling, and when my relationship became rocky, I was sad for a long time. I didn't have much enjoyment being there for school anymore.

I guess that's what you'd call love, and heartbreak.

That fun first year of college had turned into a very challenging second year, and I found myself struggling quite a lot. I was unable to get myself out of this limbo, and it truly took a toll on me.

With all the work and college stress, I began noticing 'off balance' spells more frequently and I easily got fatigued. I simply blamed all of it on the changes and stressors around me and didn't pay much attention to it. I would tell myself that I needed rest and would sleep for a couple of hours whenever I got the time. While being on the campus, I would have to walk long distances from one class to another, and that tired me out even more. It was just easier and more obvious to me at the time to point fingers at my emotional state.

When I was unable to tackle all of it together, I finally gave in to the realization that my well-being and studies were just not jiving at MSU. I was emotionally drained.

I came home. I poured my heart out to my mother, who persuaded me to finish college at a university closer to home in St. Louis. She told me that I would be able to concentrate more on my studies, and less on finances. I decided to take her up on her advice and transferred my credits to Maryville University, finishing the remainder of my two years there. Believe it or not, it was probably one of the wisest decisions I could have ever made. I straightened up my life and cut down on most of the parties. (Don't get me wrong. I still made time for a few.)

I also got a job at a Psychiatric Hospital, as it seemed mental health was on the radar for my studies. I worked and studied a lot, but by living at home, I didn't have to deal with financial stress.

My work there lasted a year, give or take; working there was very demanding, and every day was different—I never knew what to expect. It was quite the experience, but I learned so much. And even though I had the heart to work in the mental health industry, I learned that this kind of work was not quite for me. It was taxing and emotionally draining. I was pretty good about not "bringing work home" with me, but it took every ounce of emotional energy out of me when I was there. I felt I was exerting a lot of myself, and not really seeing the effects of how much of myself I poured into it all reflected back in my co-workers or the patients. It was definitely the kind of job where I had taken one step forward, but two steps back.

I took a few weeks to gather myself and look for work that I would enjoy. I buried my head in my books and focused on completing my degree. Maryville is a smaller university, which meant smaller classes compared to MSU, and you were noticed if you skipped class, so I made sure not to play hooky.

I studied very hard and am still proud of myself for the effort I put in at that time. I even made the Dean's List before graduating in December of 2010. It took me one extra semester since I had switched schools, and some of my credits didn't transfer. After I declared my major in Psychology and Sociology, I could finally figure out my future! I realized that I had the desire to work in counseling with children.

I landed a job at a preschool and worked as a teacher's assistant; I figured it would be a great place to work, considering my goals. I also had big plans to get my Masters, so I could eventually pursue counseling. I really loved working at the preschool and valued the bonds I made with the children. Working with kids was quite draining, albeit very rewarding. It felt like things were starting to fall back into my old, comfy, happy place.

It can't be good all the time, though, *right?*

The clumsiness was starting to make itself more obvious. Soon, I noticed that I had to pay extra attention to maintain my balance while walking or moving and focus to keep a steady hand. Even though the symptoms had started to become more apparent, I somehow convinced myself that everything was fine and that I didn't need to go to a doctor. Things were finally going smoothly, and I was not ready to take up another problem. I think part of the reason why I delayed the whole thing was that I wanted to feel happy for more than just one hot minute.

Looking back, the symptoms had started to appear somewhere around the age of seventeen or eighteen years old. I would notice, in a few instances or situations, that I would just suddenly trip, or feel like I had "two left feet;" while in other situations, I could maintain perfect balance. It would always take me by surprise— struggling for a few seconds before I could regain a good balance.

In the beginning, it didn't really make a lot of sense to me. My standing and walking were affected first, and I thought that, no matter what it was that was making my legs go weak and act all funny, I just needed to concentrate hard enough to keep it intact. Whatever was happening was at the forefront of my mind by this point, and I started to feel like I was constantly catching my balance. Little did I know it would end up affecting all of my body.

Even when the symptoms had really started to set in, I refused to accept the fact that something was actually wrong with me— mostly because of the nonspecificity of my symptoms. But the people around me believed something wasn't right, either. I even overheard some comments that I must be drunk or on drugs. Comments like those really gave me a punch to the gut! I felt embarrassed, but I didn't know why, and I didn't know what to do about it.

I don't really know why I never spoke to my parents about it or even told them that something didn't feel right. Was I scared? Embarrassed? Worried? Not ready to face a hard truth? I had been told by a doctor years earlier that I had "bad knees," so a part of me just figured that to be the culprit. I was trying to convince myself that my symptoms were probably just a normal thing for someone with bad knees, as though people would struggle more with balance in that case.

I guess that phase I spent convincing myself that it was nothing lasted longer than it should have. A large chunk of my struggle to come to terms with it was due to my mental state, though. I thought that if I stayed close to the walls and railings, took fewer steps, walked less, and if I used flatter shoes, I would eventually be fine. I would get over whatever it was. When my symptoms would hit me more frequently and intensely, I felt consciously safer with walls and railings, and fewer stairs to navigate.

The mental aspect must have been affecting my progress as well—this I know—because I definitely felt confident that I wouldn't trip and stumble so long as I played by the rules I had created for myself in order to feel safe; but when there was an open floor plan or lots of stairs, I panicked on the inside, which led to my losing balance right away. So I would psych myself out, in that case. Or maybe I was just aware of my limitations. It felt like my knees would lock up and I had an extremely hard time being graceful.

It often crossed my mind that I could continue to prolong getting checked out by a doctor, so long as I made sure the floor plan was how I liked it. Obviously, though, that couldn't go on forever. Just wishful thinking on my young, unsuspecting part.

My bodily changes and lack of acceptance toward whatever was happening to me made the whole condition worse. I was unable to understand. I was coping with it all alone, since I wasn't talking to anyone about it, including my parents. I wasn't avoiding anyone about it, but the more I kept my thoughts to myself, the less real it all seemed. I didn't want to talk about the clumsiness with anyone. If someone made a joke about me seeming drunk or something like that, I would quickly find a way to shrug it off and change the topic.

Even though I wasn't in this open dialogue with my parents about my clumsiness, they obviously said some things periodically to me about what they noticed. Even still, I never initiated any conversations about it with them. If they said something, I would do my best to have the conversation as quickly as possible, kind of clamped up like a shell, just waiting for it to be over. I was that immune to looking deeper into my struggles; into seeing them for what they actually were.

I was struggling on a daily basis and failed to recognize that I needed help. I truly thought that if I believed everything was fine, it somehow would be.

CHAPTER THREE

Uncertain, Vulnerable and Alone

I was prioritizing everything except for my health. I focused on college, my social life, and kept ignoring my symptoms. By the age of twenty-one, things had progressed to a point where my balance was off kilter more frequently, and those who saw me often enough had started to notice. Close relatives and friends who had seen me grow up since childhood started commenting on my balance issues—and that's when I came to realize that something may actually be wrong. The more I tripped and felt unsteady, the more I started paying attention to my problem. I began to realize that I couldn't ignore it any longer. I compared myself to others. I compared myself to my friends, who didn't have any such problems.

It was all starting to click in, to reveal itself to me. Or at least, I was finally willing to start really seeing it.

As soon as I surrendered to the realization that this clumsiness was, in fact, not normal, I decided to take matters into my own hands. I began my hunt to get to the bottom of whatever was happening. I started googling, reading articles, and carrying out extensive research, but I couldn't narrow in on anything, in particular, that could be the cause of my symptoms.

While I was at it, searching away for my solution, I got a postcard in the mail advertising two general physicians opening a new practice right by my subdivision. I jumped at the opportunity, as the general physician I usually went to was also a family friend, so I didn't really want to get his opinion on my condition. I wanted to do it purely on my own, with no one knowing that I was getting checked.

I decided to go for my first visit, all alone. When the doc asked me why I had come in, I began my story about the lack of balance I had been experiencing for a few years. The doctor asked me a few more questions and then asked me to do some walking. She noticed the slight of a drunkard gait: red flag #1. She told me to close my eyes and bring my feet together. I swayed a lot: red flag

#2. She tested my strength, which was great: no red flag there. I am sure she did more tests, but I can't remember it all. Whatever her notes and instincts told her, she referred me to an ENT specialist. I went to see him, and he thought I might have an inner ear issue, commonly known to result in balance issues.

That right there was the beginning of the many doctor visits I had to go to, in order to get to my final diagnosis. The ENT doctor did a lot of the same tests as the general physician had, and ruled out causes that had pointed to an inner ear problem. He pretty much said that he didn't know what exactly was going on with me, but that there was… something. He wanted me to go to a Neurologist next, to do further tests, because it seemed to be *something* beyond his reach.

I started to feel extremely nervous because two-for-two doctors had come up with no answers; only concerns. I had gone to these two doctors by myself, and the fact that I was unable to get answers truly frustrated and worried me. I had mixed emotions of fear, confusion, frustration, sadness, and maybe a little doubt in the healthcare providers. I mean, since they wouldn't figure out my problem, maybe there wasn't one? Maybe it was something so little, they were just overlooking it? All these feelings, combined together, really just made me feel numb. Doubt in hand, I went to the third doctor—the Neurologist. This was the third time that the same tests and procedures were being done on me. Little did I know this would come to be my new norm in my life, and soon thereafter.

They made me do a bunch of tests, which by now I've basically memorized. They are:

• Tests for mental status: They would ask me general questions, including the date, my name, etc., and I was asked to recall lists, identify objects, and even draw specific things as I was guided.

• Tests on coordination and balance: I would have to do, as I shared above, such things as place one foot before the other, bring my legs together, walk a straight line, or close my eyes while touching my nose with my finger. Similar to a sobriety test.

• Tests of the reflexes: You remember, from your younger years, going in for a checkup, and seeing the doctor bring out that small, orange-beige colored hammer? Here's where they test your responses to stimuli, by tapping on various parts of the body, such as the kneecaps, elbows, and ankles, with that little device. If the reflexes are good, the body will respond to the little hammer.

• Tests on sensation: This is what it seems. The doctor would touch my body in different parts with various instruments and items, and then ask me to define the sensations I felt, whether they felt cool, painful, warm, etc.

• Tests on the cranial nerves: The doctors asked me here to identify different smells or noises, shift my head side-to-side, or stick out my tongue while trying to talk; all to see the connection between the nerves and their affiliated organs, such as the eyes, ears, tongue, throat, etc.

• Tests on the autonomic nervous system: Where the doctor would test for regular, steady breathing, a normal heart rate and blood pressure, and a regulated body temperature[1].

At that time, when I went and saw the third doctor—the neurologist—I was surprised when he ordered an MRI of my brain. I now know that it's pretty common to administer an MRI when it comes to ruling out neurological disorders; regardless, it really made me anxious then. At that point, I hadn't been sure of whether I needed to go forward with all of this alone or actually have someone with me, by my side. Now that I was going down the line of doctors and tests, however, I asked my mom to come along. And I'm sure glad I did. She's been my rock ever since.

To be honest, I don't remember much about going to that third doctor with my mom. What I do remember is having this numb feeling come over me. I felt like I was just going to keep

[1] "Neurological Exam: MedlinePlus Medical Test." MedlinePlus, U.S. National Library of Medicine, 9 Sept. 2021, medlineplus.gov/lab-tests/neurological-exam/.

visiting different doctors without any kind of a diagnosis to show for it. There are glimpses of that day, though: I remember sitting in the waiting room with my mom before the test. I remember feeling very confined in the narrow MRI machine. Then it taking what felt like forty-five minutes to do the MRI. And finally, sitting in the waiting room while the doctor looked over the results.

This whole thing had taken a serious turn. The neurologist wanted to rule out multiple sclerosis (MS). I learned that day that the MRI was to check for lesions on the brain. I knew in my gut that I wasn't suffering from MS and that oddly calmed me down a little bit. But everything else that was going on around me really worked me up. It's a nerve-wracking place to be, waiting in the imaging center for test results with the other various cohorts. You just know that no one is there to have a good time.

At the end of the test reading, my gut feeling was right, and I did not have MS. *Thank You, Baby Jesus!* That was good news, of course, but still, I didn't get what I had come in for. The neurologist was unable to give me a proper diagnosis. Instead, he recommended that I book an appointment with a Specialty Neurologist (who I later found out specialized in genetic diseases and movement disorders) at Washington University, a wonderful research and teaching hospital in St. Louis. Dr. Matthew Harms was the one who finally gave me an answer; not the one I was looking for, but finally, I had one.

He had asked me to do all the other tests I was far too familiar with by this point, as well as some more extensive ones, as well. He was so kind and calm; yet very direct in the way he explained everything—which was honestly quite nice, just to know what he was looking for. However, it being a teaching hospital, he had a student in the room with us, so he needed to be vocal anyway. Dr. Harms seemed to have been doing this for forever, even though, to me, he'd appeared to only be in his mid-thirties. Still, I felt confident under his care. He checked my speech, muscle strength, eye movements, and reflexes and asked me to sing a musical note and hold it for as long as possible.

Even though I'd had the hammer to the knee test done before, when he did it, I felt more nervous than ever that I had no reflexes. When I'd been told I had "bad knees" years prior, I didn't have knee reflexes, but was told it wasn't a big deal; some people just don't have reflexes. This can also happen due to nerve damage, though, which I believe gave this doctor red flag #3. Dr. Harms indicated toward my nerve endings, that they were not working properly. But without definitive results, my "why's" couldn't really be answered yet. Dr. Harms decided to also perform an Electromyogram (EMG), which measures the electrical activity of muscle cells. It was quite painful, to be honest. I was in tears, and it felt like the nerve endings in my legs and feet were being electrocuted. I involuntarily kept reflexing. I didn't know that this journey I had set foot on would bring its answers through so much pain.

After all this testing, Dr. Harms shortlisted three conditions and told me that he was very sure that it was one of the three. He added that, to get the final diagnosis, we needed some more in-depth blood work (i.e., genetics tests).

I can't exactly remember what the other two diagnoses were that he had written down, but Friedreich's Ataxia (FA) was by far the scariest one. Of course, I went home and researched myself down a rabbit hole in all three of these conditions. FA had a worse prognosis than the others. All I read across the computer screen were sentences that included words like "wheelchair," "dependent," "life-shortening," "no treatments or cure," and the like. Quite nerve-wracking, to say the least.

That night was horrible for me, and I was scared to death about having this disease. The other two conditions that were part of his list had a simple treatment course and not as many harsh words to describe the prognosis. I hoped and prayed so hard that it was one of the lesser ones, even though my gut was telling me—quite loudly—that it was FA.

I went back in on New Year's Eve of 2009 to get the bloodwork done, and then waited for about two weeks before hearing anything. Sometime in January of 2010, the final diagnosis was in. I wasn't sure if I was ready to get the answer, though. After what I had read online, I was truly scared and was not sure how I would handle the truth.

I remember that day like it was yesterday; the day my doctor called me to break the news of my diagnosis. My parents and I sat around the table with the phone on speaker so we all could hear:

"I have some good news and some bad news," said the doctor.

Oh shit, what is it?! I could barely speak.

"The bad news is that you have Friedreich's Ataxia," Dr. Harms began to explain.

My head literally screamed a big, roaring, deafening *Whaaaat?!*

When I first heard it, I didn't know how to react. I think I was in shock. The worst of all possibilities was *actually* happening to me. I had no tears, no nothing yet. I was still processing. I wasn't feeling angry then. I was in complete disbelief. I completely spaced out and could only think about how miserable the rest of my life was going to be.

"The good news is, your progression rate is really slow. You will notice yourself declining at quite a slow rate," he continued.

But that sort of news is like hearing: "If nothing kills you sooner, then FA will be your deathbed; only, slow and difficult, where your body will fail you and you will have no motor control." That's intense, I know, but I can't imagine many people taking this information lightly at first.

The doctor continued to tell me how there was no treatment or cure and that I needed to visit his office so that he could explain everything in detail for me to understand, so that I could be more prepared for life ahead.

You know how it happens in the movies, when you see someone being diagnosed with cancer or something, where the sad music cues as they zone out, while the doctor and everything else becomes background noise? Well, that's exactly what happened at that moment. I can't quite remember the melody… but when I finally zoned back in, I mustered up the strength to ask him one of the things I cared deeply about: "Will I be able to have kids?"

I had dreamt of having my own family, with a loving husband and a whole lot of kids; so, naturally, that was very important to me. Even at twenty-two.

To my relief, he replied, "It is very much possible to have children, have a healthy marriage, succeed in your career with FA, and do much, much more."

That right there gave me so much hope. I felt the blood begin to flow through my veins again. I wasn't dead on the inside anymore. I knew it would all be challenging and test every ounce of patience I possessed, but that it was possible. At least it was all still *possible*.

That was all I needed to hear.

CHAPTER FOUR

What Is Friedreich's Ataxia?

Depending on the web page or book you read, or who you talk with, Friedreich's Ataxia can sound divergent in regards to its symptoms and severity; so at first, it could sound either like some super random disease with unfortunate symptoms, or else, as though I am crippled and dying tomorrow.

Friedreich's Ataxia (FA) really is a debilitating, life-shortening, degenerative neuro-muscular disorder[2]. At least, that's how it is defined. For me, it feels mostly like a challenge—a cloud looming over my life—or like one long, bad day that just won't end.

Friedreich's Ataxia was first identified by the German physician Nikolaus Friedreich in 1863; however, it wasn't until 1876 that he articulated the hereditary nature of the disorder. Over one hundred years later, in 1996, the discovery of the genetic defect underlying FA was found, at which point it was officially labeled as a genetic disorder. Before this defective gene was uncovered to be the underlying reason for the disease, the diagnosis was based upon symptoms only[3]. I'm certainly thankful for how far science has come in its level of awareness around FA in recent years.

FA is quite a rare condition that primarily affects the nervous system and the heart. It isn't caused by the particular actions of a person, nor is it infectious. Don't worry—we can still hold hands and you won't catch anything from me!

It is, in easy terms, an inherited disorder caused by a defective gene that can be transferred from one generation to the next.

---

[2] FARA - Home, www.curefa.org/.

[3] Jörg B. Shultz and Massimo Pandolfo, 2013.

This infamous defective gene is called the frataxin (FXN) gene, basically because the mutation of this gene (which causes FA) limits the production of frataxin, an essential protein that operates in the mitochondria of our cells. Mitochondria, in case you can't recall your cell drawings and breakdowns from Biology class, serve as the energy production factory of the cell; and frataxin, as a protein, moves iron through the cell to create iron-sulfur clusters that help produce this energy for each cell, and thus for the body[4]. Without frataxin, the mitochondria are ineffective, thus causing faulty energy production for the cells of the body.

Of course, I'm no doctor, but it only makes sense to me that an easy fix for someone with FA would be to give them injections of frataxin. *I mean… right?!* Since frataxin is the protein I am lacking, it seems simple to me to just put some of this frataxin (natural or synthetic) into a syringe and then inject this juice into my body. Sort of how a diabetic needs their insulin.

I know the textbook-like interpretation of my disorder in this chapter may have taken you on a one-way trip to Snoozeville— like, *What are you getting us into, here, Erin?!*—so thank you for being patient with me! All in all, Friedreich's Ataxia is super, duper rare. It's both rare to inherit it and rare to know about it. It's so rare, it's shitty: shitty to get, and shitty to live with. But still—you can have *normalcy*. And I think that it's important for the world to know this—about those with FA, and about me. *We can have normalcy.* So let us all take off our ignorance caps and burn them, as we level up in our understanding of disabilities and capabilities!

---

[4] Moore, Charles. "Converting Skin Cells into Sensory Neurons Could Offer Therapeutic…" Friedreich's Ataxia News, 29 Dec. 2014.

I for one kept severely quiet about my illness at first, mostly because of the generalized tone of depression that would always surround disabilities in common society. But normalcy is possible—if not preferable. Those of us with disabilities, yes, may *need* to be treated with a different type of care than most capable humans; however, I'm pretty close to positive that no one with a disability wants to be pitied. Not a one of us wishes to be looked down upon, or as though our experience of being a person is in any way *less than* that of an able-bodied person.

After I was first diagnosed, when I would think about sharing my diagnosis with others, or talking about it, my throat would just about close up. I would experience this overwhelming sense of shame around having a disease. So after my diagnosis, I just waited, and waited…. I kept it to myself. I was nervous to be seen by others in any way *less than*, pitiable, or somehow damaged.

Making my disease a reality meant that the things I wanted in life may be more challenging to acquire than what I was prepared for. Once I let it in, I'd have to deal with the limitations head-on. It would have to become a part of my official story, a part of my reality—a part of *me*.

Once I made the switch and came out with it, though, it did feel like a relief, and it felt good to educate others on something that needed to be recognized. I started to learn the truth about having an illness, and began slowly to foster my own version of how the disability would be woven into the story of my life.

When I stopped hiding my diagnosis, I certainly felt less embarrassed and secluded. I learned, over time, how it's actually much easier for people to understand and relate to me when I am open and honest about it all. I started to realize that it was kind of like killing two birds with one stone because I felt more confident in being real and open, and it was enlightening to educate people about a rare and unique disease they didn't otherwise know about.

So now… back to the basics: FA is inherited through what's called an autosomal recessive manner, meaning that individuals with FA have two mutated or abnormal copies of the FXN gene. This means both biological parents must be a carrier of the disease for a child to be affected. So, yes, my mom and dad are carriers of the abnormalities of the FXN gene, but thankfully, exhibit neither signs nor symptoms.

When I said that Friedreich's Ataxia was *rare* earlier—it is estimated that 1 in 100 people are carriers, although carriers do not exhibit any of the symptoms of FA. So it's not that uncommon to be a carrier—you might even be!

Worldwide, though, about 1 in 50,000 individuals are affected by FA, making it the most prevalent in a category of associated disorders called *hereditary ataxias*. "Ataxia" means lack of order. There are a number of types of Ataxias with a number of causes. Friedreich's Ataxia is one type of this condition, and, to me, it is by far the *sexiest* of all the ataxias!

A carrier parent of FA will have one mutated FXN allele and one normal FXN allele. Because each child gets one of the mother's genes and one of the father's genes in this location, there are four possible combinations of the genes passed down to the child, or a 25% chance that the child will have FA.

I *definitely* pulled the short end of the stick on that one!

Though, a part of me wasn't by any means surprised by my luck of the draw. I've always considered myself to be the type of person who would have to carry the weight of something odd. I have a massive extended family, and yet I'm the only one with FA, or even a physical disability for that matter…. Like, what are the actual chances?!

I constantly am battling with inner qualms of *Why me?* I don't want to feel like a victim, but at times, I do. I know it sounds a bit harsh, but then I figure there's gotta be a great purpose behind my being chosen to have this. I like the idea that when you're served lemons, you're just being asked to make some lemonade—to turn the shitty things on your plate into something good.

And speaking of turning lemons into lemonade, I'm going to try to spin some more factual stuff regarding FA into knowledge gold. This is the stuff you [should've] learnt in science class in high school when you were doodling in your notebook, instead.

Normally, the FXN gene will cause your body to produce up to 33 copies of a specific DNA sequence. In people with Friedreich's Ataxia, this sequence may repeat 66 to over 1,000 times. When production of this DNA sequence spirals out of control like this, severe damage to the brain's cerebellum (the part of the brain that controls balance and coordination) and the spinal cord can result. Remember, this is the part of the brain that assists in coordination, not thoughts. I'm pretty sure some people instantly connect mental challenges with being disabled, but this is a wrong assumption.

The signs and symptoms of FA can include a loss of coordination, or ataxia, in areas of the body where movement and control work together; scoliosis, or a curvature of the spine; fatigue; slurred speech, vision impairment and hearing loss; muscle weakness and loss of muscle mass; diabetes; and serious heart conditions such as hypertrophic cardiomyopathy and arrhythmias[5]. These symptoms are not present in all individuals with FA, however. Diabetes, for example, occurs in only about 10-20% of individuals with FA.

The progressive loss of coordination and muscle strength that comes with this disorder generally leads to motor incapacitation, or the full-time use of a wheelchair. Many young people who are diagnosed with FA will require mobility aids such as a cane, walker, or wheelchair by their teens or early twenties. Most people experience the onset of their symptoms somewhere between the ages of five and eighteen. Adult or late onset FA is less common, making up less than twenty-five percent of diagnosed individuals, and can occur anytime during adulthood[6].

I was diagnosed shortly after turning twenty-two, but FA showed glimpses in my late teens. And thankfully for me, many of the hardships of FA, I do not have. At this time, having been diagnosed over ten years ago now, I do experience the obvious lack of balance and coordination, slightly slurred speech, and fatigue—I'll take a caffeine IV, please!

I also go through lack of sensation and circulation, which at times can really suck. It's mostly in my lower legs and feet; they're typically seen sporting the blue-and-purple look. I don't necessarily like the way it looks, but I've come to terms that it's just another unfortunate side effect of FA, and have learned to control what I can by keeping my lower appendages warm with socks, slippers or blankets, and keeping my dogs elevated, soaking up the warm, natural Vitamin D from the front porch.

---

[5] "Team Kendall: About Friedreich's Ataxia." Team Kendall, www.teamkendall.org/aboutfa.

[6] "What Is FA." Voices of Friedreich's Ataxia (FA), voicesoffa.org/what-is-fa/.

I probably can withstand heat and hot showers more than the average Joe. But I'm also far too familiar with feeling cold and I am sure you'll hear me say, "Brrrr, it's chilly," often enough. I know I've probably had the water on too hot a time or two, because I've come out of the shower looking like a flaming hot Cheeto or a lobster, as though I'd soaked in the sun too long. My Irish skin can't take it, but my Italian blood is saying, *Oh yeahh*. The warmer the better, in my book!

I honestly dream about moving south, though. I plan out how I'll live and how it will feel: I imagine living in very southern Florida. Like *The Keys*. It's always so warm there, so *hot*, which is exactly how I want it! Yet it's breezy, and I love being close to the ocean so I can always hear the crashing of waves—windows and doors are always open in my home. As much as I'd love family, especially Eli, to live close by, I picture myself living alone and making friends with the locals. And I have a great vacation spot which I can imagine family and friends will want to come visit. But—maybe… I'm not alone? Maybe my dreamboat of a long-lost love is with me?

I picture starting many mornings out on my patio and writing. Whether just to get words off my chest, work on my blog, or possibly to write another book.

I live close by to a few eateries where I become a regular. I probably always eat outside and watch the water. Hear the seagulls and toads ribbiting in nearby swamps. Ah… and the crickets!

I probably don't go on the beach much because even those "sand wheelchairs" made specifically for the sand are hard to maneuver. I'll be as close as I can be, without being on the sand.

I'll take tons of boat rides because nothing is more peaceful than being on the water with the wind blowing fast and the sun beating down. And a clear view of palm trees. *Ahhhhh…* The taste of eating fruits and vegetables from a farmers' market. Freshly squeezed juice, sipping it on my patio. Feeling completely zen. At peace. No hostility in paradise.

So much of my life is about managing my comfort. I dream of a life where I simply get to kick back, relax, and have my needs and preferences all met. Though, I guess many of us could agree to this definition of paradise!

In stark contrast to this daydream, a very real and somewhat newer nightmare of a symptom I've been experiencing lately is choking. It doesn't happen often, but enough to catch me off guard and be a true nuisance as I cough to clear my throat. It happens only with liquids I drink, my salvia, or certain foods like cereal, nuts, and crackers—pretty much the kinds of foods that produce a lot of "crumbs." It may be the only thing I am self-conscious about when I'm out and about now, since it definitely draws a lot of stares—there's nothing subtle about hacking your brains out. Plus, it's scary trying to catch your breath and feeling short of air. I've learned to just keep coughing until I clear it or try to concentrate on breathing through my nose. So don't be alarmed and run over to give me the Heimlich Maneuver or make a scene if you see me in this state; just let me cough in peace.

And then just one more symptom I've come to know, which is extremely irritating, is something known as Nystagmus, where my eyes freak out in these uncontrollable, repetitive shifting movements, really fast-like. Although I rarely experience these "jerky movements," it does happen from time to time. When I concentrate on an object or read something on the TV, I lose that focus sometimes and my eyes jerk around and I have to concentrate and breathe to refocus them.

There is no cure or overall treatment for Friedreich's Ataxia, but treatments for its cardiac symptoms are available, as well as corrective surgery for scoliosis and foot curvatures, and treatable measures for diabetes. Many therapies, tips and measures are encouraged, as they can assist in managing symptoms and make life more enjoyable overall. But the biggest joy of all would be to be able to walk, run and dance the night away. I know I can speak for the FA community on this one!

I've done, for example, plenty of physical, occupational and speech therapies to help reduce my symptoms and relearn everyday tasks; but with the progression of the disease, unfortunately, the tasks need to be altered every so often to accommodate the changes.

The progression of my disease, for me, has looked like this:

The symptoms started subtly. I guess my first memories of its effects would be of not being able to run as fast or go down stairs as quickly as I once could. I'd catch myself from feeling off balance and really liked the idea of railings to hold onto, of course. It took a year or two until the imbalance progressed and then my upper body coordination started to kick in negatively. I was spilling while walking with a full glass of water. It was so weird to me because I felt like I was always holding it sturdy, but I guess my walking was a little off and was making it hard for me to use my upper body as gracefully as I had before.

With some trial and error, I began to realize that it was smartest for me to do the more laborious stuff earlier in the day, when I had the most energy. When I had school, work, or social events later in the evening or at night, I had a harder time with my balance and coordination. That's when I'd really have to assess the floor plan to see what I was in for. Could I wear heels? Or flat shoes?

Did I need more caffeine, to give me more energy? Could I drink alcohol without falling over? Where was the bathroom? And the front door? Can I avoid stairs? If not, are there railings?

My assessment of the floor plan started early on with FA and is still a thing for me today, with just a bit more to be aware of: Handicap bathrooms. Ramps. Elevators. Parking.

The hardest part about the disease, for me, is the progression. I find myself having to reaccept and come to terms with my disability all over again whenever my symptoms progress.

I don't think I can narrow down my *first* memory of FA showing its subtle colors, quite; but I do remember, during the last year or two of high school, noticing that I was going down stairs differently than before. My high school had three floors, so it was constant to go up and down the stairs all day long, but by senior year I just felt better holding onto the railing while going down the stairs. I remember thinking, *My knees must really be giving out on me,* and just attributed the imbalance to the knee problem.

I did become more and more aware of this as that year went by, and absolutely hated that I was becoming more reliant on railings. However, the more I paid attention to this "problem," I also began to recognize that there were times where I felt completely comfortable going down staircases without the railings. I was able to go down stairs without a railing whenever the walls weren't too far apart and there were less than five steps—and the lesser the better for the amount of people who could possibly see me, too.

That mental aspect of it all played a huge role in how well I could walk. If I was overthinking it, or got nervous, my whole body would shake, and I would lose my necessary semblance of control over it. I feared physically hurting myself from a fall. More than that, though, I didn't want to embarrass myself. Since I didn't really know yet what was going on with me, I didn't want anyone confronting me that they thought something was wrong with me. I wouldn't have known how to handle it.

An event where perhaps more people had a perplexed look directed towards me was at my high school graduation. With hundreds of people's eyes on me and nothing to hold onto while I walked and stood out in the open, I got nervous, thinking, *What if my knees give out and I fall?* I nervously started shaking, and I'm sure that may have led a lot of people to question what was going on with me. I wasn't openly talking about it all at the time, though, so I always just found a way to deflect the attention away from the topic.

During college, it became more apparent to me because walking the campus to and from class felt to me like I was hiking for miles. My body felt tense every time I had to walk. I really needed to put effort into walking steadily, and all the while I felt like, *This should be second nature.*

Maybe the alcohol lessened the tense feeling I had, or the anxiety circling me, but I always felt better at parties where drinking was involved. Obviously, if I drank too much, then like anyone would, I staggered. There were times when I said, "Fuck it, I'm drinking and partying all night!" But most times, I knew my limit and cut myself off before I was staggering too much.

In my freshman year of college, my friend Megan from high school was my roommate. We had a room on the second floor of our dormitory which was called 'Freddy' for short. We were in our room trying to fall asleep but we kept freaking each other out about a ghost in our room. We kept hearing little things and we were convinced we were being haunted. We said to one another that, on the count of three, we'd jump out of our beds, unlock our door and run down the hall. We did that, and screamed, "There's a ghost in our room!" all the way down the hall, holding hands.

I remember thinking how hard it was to run. I tried so hard but it felt impossible to get my legs going that quick. I was holding Megan's hand, so I am pretty sure she was just pulling me to try and keep me at her pace. But it felt so strange that I couldn't control my speed. It was like all the instincts were going off in my brain, but to get the rest of my body to move at a quick pace was a failing attempt. The signals were short circuiting, and sparks were flying—but no dice.

CHAPTER FIVE

Physical Therapy

I started Physical Therapy (PT) in January of 2012. I had been diagnosed for a couple of years by this point, but had kept going independently, doing what I could to "treat" myself—whether by holding walls, railings, people's arms, or hiding whatever symptoms I possibly could.

As much as I fought against and ignored making any sort of therapy a reality, I ultimately surrendered and began the process of welcoming in the other ends and variables of this disease. This doesn't mean I ever liked it—and honestly, I still don't—but in order to function independently, I needed to learn to try and adapt to assistive devices, as well as continuously accept therapy treatments to support my performance of tasks as symptoms continued to progress.

I have taken part in multiple sessions of Physical Therapy since 2012. The initial visits of each start-up are more of seeing what actions I can perform and how well I can do them with a goal in mind to be reached. A question I am always asked by my physical therapist is: "What's your goal?"

My immediate response is, "To walk without assistance," and as many times as I've been to Physical Therapy, that's always my answer; however, it is pretty farfetched, and I usually back it up with a smaller goal so it actually seems like I am making reasonable strides as I move along. It may be something like building my endurance, learning tasks to make transferring from sitting to standing more fluid, or working on my strength so I can feel more confident standing and walking without buckling or toppling over.

When I welcomed PT in January of 2012, I also began the hunt for an assisted device; after trying out some walkers, canes and crutches, a walker seemed to be the best fit, but it was a weird and overwhelming process to discern through. When envisioning a 'walker,' my mind would snap to the image of an eighty-year-old. I was in my early twenties at the time—that surely couldn't be what was next on my life list! It took some time to become confident in strutting the frame, and I quickly had to get over the "woe is me" attitude, as I needed my mind and body working in sync in order to get the whole walker thing down.

It is very important to have the mind and body working together, because the more my brain tells my body negative things, it surely isn't going to give a friendly welcome to a walker. I was learning a whole new way to walk, transfer to sit and stand, handle a curb and steps, and everything else I needed to know to move through my world. I was learning all the basics like a one-year-old does, but with a walker. Even though I was doing my best to surrender to a mobility aid, it was hard and scary and, frankly, heartbreaking. My capabilities were getting tougher and at some point, they could be stripped away to a point of total dependency.

I don't think I will ever be okay or fully content with losing the abilities FA has and will continue to take from me.

I never knew how much it really entailed, to simply *walk*.

Walking is something that most do every day, without even thinking about it. It seems very simple and straightforward. You just put one foot in front of the other... and you move. But walking takes more than just moving your feet and legs. You use your core, glutes, back and hips which coordinate in a certain motion to propel you forward. The way your limbs and muscles move is in a coordinated alternating pattern, and as FA does not like to make any kind of movement graceful, walking becomes problematic. Losing something vital—not only to walk, but proper leg movement to help do other tasks—is a very difficult thing to cope with. It definitely requires some mourning before you're able to get yourself back out in the world again. It's a big, deep, profound loss.

I vividly remember my very first visit to PT and couldn't believe how sore I was just from moving from sit to stand to walk to laying down. This was a huge wakeup call that I needed more movement in my life and couldn't let FA keep me down or hold me back. PT was a great thing, in hindsight. Yet I probably wouldn't have started physical therapy at that time, had I not fallen on the driveway that day with Sylvia.

Blessings in disguise, for sure.

When I got the walker I needed, it played such an important part in my life, so my friend came up with a name for it—*Sylvia! It's a girl! It needs a name if it's always going to hang out, right?!* Sylvia was one of those silver walkers—See how she got her name?!—that most may relate a Granny to using. I tried out those fancy rollator walkers with the seat in the middle but the wheels on those walkers move in every direction and I find it hard to glide and walk smoothly with them. I never understood how ataxia patients liked the rollator; with our coordination, we are all over the place, and those wheels don't help any. But different strokes for different folks, I guess.

Now that Sylvia was an official part of the family, I used a lot of what I learned from PT to maneuver around. It's much different and more difficult to do everything on your own versus having a therapist by your side, practicing at a facility designed to be accessible. The real world is much easier for able-bodied people to maneuver around, so the run-ins of hills, grass, stairs, cracks, and long distances opened up new obstacles for me. Those challenges probably will remain during my lifetime; it's inevitable, but adapting to them is super important.

I started using a wheelchair more and more around 2016-2017. I had used a wheelchair for long distances like airports, the zoo, "walks" at the park, etc. before then, but started using it more at this point because of having recently broken my rib in the fall.

Quite a painful bone to break in your body, because no position is comfortable as it heals; even breathing hurts! Anyway, walking with the walker was not only painful, but I was still a bit shaken up and nervous to start walking without falling again, so I felt more comfortable relying on a wheelchair. I had just been using a generic, previously owned wheelchair from a facility like a Goodwill as a mobility aid, so it wasn't exactly equipped for my body; it was a bit bulky, but I made do.

This incident allowed me to get more acquainted with the wheelchair, until I realized I was starting to feel pretty dependent upon it to get around. And once I was sitting more, I needed to *again* sign up for PT and OT, to learn more tasks in taking care of myself from a wheelchair-user point of view. It truly is exhausting, when I think about it. When I compare it with the way things had used to be.

This round of therapy was a lot of transferring in and out of the wheelchair using a safe technique. Learning how to manipulate curbs from the chair without toppling out. And getting a lot of exercise in, with being out of the wheelchair, so I could keep my legs and core strong. I use a manual wheelchair, so I use my arms to propel and my goodness, do they get tired!

I've learned some tips in PT on the best times and ways to wheel myself around, and also found that I do not like using foot pedals on the chair to rest my feet on. I rather like to take them off, so I can use my feet to help with propelling and moving. I look kind of like I'm doing a walking motion, only sitting down. It helps to give my arms a rest so they're not working so hard for the rest of my body.

Some of the exercises I'd perform in PT would include coordination exercises, or gait training, which are recommended for patients with Ataxia to facilitate proprioception, or a sense of motion, position, and balance—something which is often lost in FA.

Testing my proprioception is quite the challenge. The second I close my eyes, if standing, I sway and more often than not, fall over. Same if there is no light. The darkness and the closing of the eyes make it quite impossible for me to maintain balance (hence the broken rib). I also have a hard time telling where my limbs are in space. For example: I am sitting, eyes closed, and someone moves my toe upwards or downwards, and I must guess which direction they're moving it, and I struggle. I can feel that my toe is being moved, but I have a difficult time sensing its position. It's a strange concept; feeling it, but being unsure of where it is.

It's quite the challenge to do balance exercises on my own, but when I used Sylvia, I was able to do an exercise of simply standing and letting go of the walker to test my balance. With the progression of the disease, I now use my wheelchair to get around, so practicing balance on my own is tough. I feel safer practicing when someone is around to assist me, but that isn't always the case. That isn't always available to me. But I still need to move and stretch and exercise when I'm on my own, so I'll do a lot of floor work.

I can also test my balance by kneeling and engaging my core to keep me upright as long as I can hold it. I like to say that the core is the motherboard of the body. Keeping it strong and intact is super important for being able to keep the rest of the body moving the best you can.

The core also helps with sitting balance, which may seem to be of little importance, but ataxia does not help keep me steady while sitting, so if I'm moving my arms or any part of the body for that matter, it's a free-for-all. With a weak core and a progressed ataxia, swaying the upper body and not having the control or coordination to keep the trunk still and upright is a true problem for some. I've seen FA wheelchair users even use a seatbelt, so they don't sway out of their chair. Back support is also needed for most; maybe not in the beginning stages of FA, but as it progresses, back support is more often utilized. Personally, as the day goes by, my back and neck start to feel as if I've moved heavy furniture for hours; I'm sore, and I need to rest my back and neck.

When I do my floor exercises, you can catch me laying on my back with my legs up on the couch for a good fifteen minutes. The flat, hard surface feels so good and releases a lot of tension. I use that short time to meditate, which I feel is equally as important as exercise. Meditation really helps me gather my thoughts, which seem to bounce around my head and can cause me to get overwhelmed. Since I'm already on the floor, I like to get in some yoga to really stretch my neck and back and incorporate some balance and strength exercises from sitting, kneeling, or even laying down. Yoga really is a "one-man-band." It helps to relieve so much of the tightness and constricted feelings from using the wheelchair. In yoga I can stretch, move my body more freely, be flexible and take deep breaths that feel so easy to inhale and exhale through.

Even though it's safer for me to use a wheelchair, it is very uncomfortable to just sit all day long! Our bodies are not meant to be sitting all day, every day. It's rough on the back and the pelvis and it doesn't promote quality circulation through the body. To be blunt, it can cause many health problems with the heart, blood pressure, and just poor engagement of certain muscles. Plus, do you know how difficult it is to do *everything* from a seated position?! *IT'S HARD AF!* I can't tell you the many times I've tried to stand up from the couch and envisioned myself just walking to the bathroom. *Ohhh, what a dream.* When I used Sylvia, I thankfully could walk around, but once I started needing the wheelchair, I would just transition from one seat to the other.

I do not enjoy having to be dependent on a wheelchair.

In addition to yoga, it's important that I incorporate whatever vigorous exercise I can to get my heart pumping faster, blood circulating and to build muscle tone so my muscles don't atrophy (loss of muscle tissue = weak and flabby looking). I have a stationary bike and a squat machine for some cardio and to get my legs and ankles moving to gain strength.

In addition to doing my exercises at home, I work out at a gym, Fitzmaurice Performance, with a trainer, Lisa, and before Lisa, her brother, Shawn. It's a family-owned, private gym that shines in athlete training, personal training, and group workouts. Pre Covid-19, I was going twice a week, from the beginning of 2014. Since the pandemic, I missed six months there, and once I continued, I had to cut down due to the occupancy protocols and other injuries life threw at me.

As stated before, I feel more comfortable doing most of my exercises with someone else, so I absolutely love my time with Lisa. She and her brother have helped me tremendously in tweaking things so that I can engage my exercises appropriately. Whether holding me upright, stabilizing my uncoordinated limbs, or having me lean against a wall, I get it done. I surprise myself often, but you never know your limits until you push yourself towards them.

We work on it all: Strength and balance training. I use free weights, dumbbells, the barbell, T.R.X. bands, a stationary bike, the Power Plate, and whatever floor work Lisa has up her sleeve. Planks and sit-ups are a must, whether I am there or at home. I gotta keep that core strong, and plus who doesn't want abs?! I can, even with my symptoms, get a full-body workout in, with a little creativity. It is *for real* possible to get the full effects of working out when movements are tweaked to one's ability. Never say, "I can't." Seriously—or else Shawn will have you do ten extra reps of something.

I was pointed in the direction of Fitzmaurice Performance to see Shawn because my Physical Therapist at the time had recommended I continue some exercise after PT to keep the momentum going. One of her patients had found Shawn to continue his own exercise, and so once I got word of it, I tracked Shawn down, dove into sharing with him all about FA and the goals I had hoped to accomplish, and he was very welcoming to me as I started my journey at Fitzmaurice Performance. After months of working with Shawn, he moved out of Missouri, and I was gifted his sister, Lisa, as my new trainer. Lisa has been my trainer for a little over five years, and she has not only kept me in shape but has become a great friend and supporter, too.

On top of PT, I've also introduced Occupational Therapy (OT) and Speech Therapy into my life. I began OT back when I'd started PT in 2012, and in sum, it's about learning new ways to take care of myself independently. In 2012, I was introducing a walker for mobility, so I needed to learn how to cook, wash dishes, do laundry, shower, get dressed... all the basics, but from a new perspective. If I could lean on the counter to wash dishes, it was doable—so long as it was under ten minutes, as my back, legs and feet would hurt thereafter from the pressure of standing.

Laundry was tricky when the clothes or towels were ready to come out of the dryer, to be folded and put away. I'd typically throw them in a laundry basket, but the challenge was getting the basket to my bed or couch so I could sit and fold them. Don't forget, I was using a walker at this point, so my hands were busy holding onto it. With my thinking very much operating outside of the box, I found I could kick the basket as I took steps with the walker. When there's a will, there is surely a way!

When it came to cooking, that was pretty tricky because I was typically using the stove or oven with lots of heat and could burn myself if not super careful. In OT, therapy was just kind of about showing the ways to lean on counters and where not to lean, how to bend over cautiously so that I wouldn't fall face first into the oven, as well as training me to take small breaks to sit while something was being stovetop cooked. Honestly, I usually just winged it, and did what I could at the time. It's not always realistic to incorporate what is taught in therapy to use at home; the placement of appliances and counter heights are always different than at the facility.

There were a lot of *Hail Mary*'s said when I cooked and many prayers I wouldn't burn myself—I am of course happy I didn't have a kitchen accident, but I wouldn't necessarily recommend winging it like I did!

My biggest help in Occupational Therapy was practicing my fine motor skills, like dexterity and strength in the wrists and fingers to help with the simple tasks of getting dressed with zippers and buttons. Sure, it sounds very simple, but these are the tasks that become so hard and taxing with FA. Especially writing. My handwriting was showing very small signs of declination and it took lots of effort to get the writing motion to be clear. I still had legible handwriting, but the speed of writing was slower and I just felt exhausted trying to keep up and take lots of notes. Holding the pen properly while gripping it is a whole process in itself. I couldn't believe I was needing tips on how to write; I couldn't believe I was being taught what a four-year-old is taught!

Speech Therapy wasn't introduced right when I started PT and OT, but I have done two or three rounds of it over the past six years. I want to say that I first started it when I noticed my speech beginning to slur a bit. This was something I knew could eventually happen, as it's a common side effect of FA, but it was another thing I had to mourn the loss of; and it sucked and still does.

Because this is progressive, I'm constantly reminded of how something so simple like talking is a full-time push for me. I am lucky my speech hasn't declined to the point of being unintelligible, but I do have to make sure my voice is strong and make my words count. When I talk, I feel it is unjust that I have to try so hard. And then it reminds me of just how hard I'm always working—just to keep up with past versions of myself. Watching myself fall apart, while doing everything I can to hold it all together.

So then, how is it fair that someone who has to make just being alive—talking, walking, swallowing, cooking, writing—a job, is also told that they should also work a job and have a career like everyone else? I hear this from people all the time. I hear from different organizations, "Oh, we can definitely place you in a job you can handle," or, "Look at other people with FA, MS, Muscular Dystrophy, etc. that work. You can too!"

So in turn, I feel shame for not working, but I choose to put my energy, instead, into raising my kid and volunteering for disability events. I couldn't fathom working and balancing being a mom *and* navigating my disease. I am already exhausted, so I've found acceptance in having simple things and a happy and healthy kid! Although a house of our own would be very awesome, I humbly can say: "I'm very thankful for what I have."

Some with FA strive to work and do whatever it takes to have a job, but what if I'm spent just from keeping myself upright and not falling to the ground when I sneeze? Or I need to rest my voice after chatting with a friend after they've had a bad day? Or my words are slurring more and more, the more I'm explaining Eli's math homework to him? And my hand is tired, and my writing isn't legible from writing practice math equations with Eli?

I've accepted the misfortunes of FA, but it surely doesn't mean I like them. I would rather walk than be in a wheelchair. I'd rather type on a computer than my phone. I'd rather talk for hours without slurring my words. I'd rather play soccer with my son than watch. I'd rather drive with my feet than my hands. I'd rather reach everything in the kitchen than ask for help. I'd rather enter through the front door with stairs than have to go through the back. I'd rather have any job I wanted, rather than finding something I can do from a chair that doesn't require coordination.

If it wasn't for my extreme positivity, my life could be very sad and depressing. FA is a very tough diagnosis, and it is exhausting to not allow it to overcome me.

As far as speech—my first encounter with someone calling me out about it was the year before I was even diagnosed with FA. That would have made me twenty-one and I was, at the time, visiting another state when I came across some people from Georgia. As we were talking, their southern drawl was very obvious and I made a comment on how thick their accent was, when they said that my Midwestern accent was like nothing they had ever heard before. I shrugged it off, thinking they just figured I had a strange accent or was drinking a few too many beers. *I didn't feel tipsy at all though…?*

One of them eventually said, "I know what it is! You're enunciating *every* word!"

I'd obviously had no idea I was doing that, but I guess my mind was off in left field, distracting me from how much effort I was already putting in to keep face. I am pretty sure I gave a perplexed look and shrugged off their assumptions about me "talking funny."

To this day, I am still understood when speaking, with the occasional, "What did you say? Repeat yourself." For me, the speaking changes were something I couldn't ignore and so I wanted to accept what help I could. My neurologist recommended and wrote an order for me to begin speech therapy, where I basically had to practice a bunch of words and sentences, both at therapy and for homework, to work on sounding clearer. It helped at the time I guess, but as time went on, I gradually stopped practicing as much. I just deal with it now and have learned to use the energy of talking for the right times. I'm a social person who has a lot to say, so it's definitely been a learning curve, cutting back on the talking. But it's also a good thing to just listen. I take the moments for gratitude wherever they surface; wherever I sift through and find them.

My second round of speech therapy went on while I was starting to have more difficulty with choking; when drinks or salvia felt like they were "going down the wrong pipe." As I shared earlier, this was a symptom that didn't come on for years after my diagnosis, but when it did, it was the scariest one, to think I could aspirate and have liquids or food sucked down into my lungs. But basically, I'd just choke and cough a lot until I cleared it out, if I did.

The domino effect, before I started this second round of speech therapy, was initially to go and see a throat and swallowing specialist so they could gage how well my throat muscles and vocal cords were working. It was not a pleasant experience, by any means—for, the doctor sent a small camera up my nose which would land in the back of my throat, from where he could then see everything on his monitor screen. I gag just thinking about it! *Yech!*

There was nothing the doctor could do for me, really, at this point, besides recommending some throat exercises to strengthen what I could control. I was taught how to strengthen my throat muscles by blowing into some weird instrument thing, amongst other exercises. My homework was to practice those at home twice a day, which again fizzled off after a few weeks because, well, I guess I wasn't mentally committed to keeping them up.

In addition to my homework, I was sent in separately for a swallowing test. The gist of this was to see what foods and liquids were troublesome for me to swallow. The doctors watched me swallow after propping me up next to this X-ray machine which allowed them to watch my throat muscles do "what they should." I started off with thicker foods like pudding, and worked my way to crackers, and different consistencies of liquids. Of course, nothing alarming would pop up while being watched like a hawk with all the medical professionals in the room, so the best they could suggest at that point was for me to go to speech therapy to learn better techniques on swallowing.

This is what began the second go at speech therapy. I learned the tuck and swallow technique, which works wonders—though it is also unlikely that I always want to do it. It's a technique where you tuck your chin to your chest and swallow to help yourself from choking. Or else there's the hard swallow technique, where you do exactly what it sounds like: swallow hard, to make sure you get it all down. Another great technique, although neither one totally resonates for me to do all the time. It actually takes more time and energy to do this with every swallow than to simply rest into allowing my swallow to be what it is. Making the most of it. I do know that it's safer with the exercises, I just have trouble doing this consistently. Maybe one day I'll get it down pat! Or maybe my body just doesn't like the forced, extraneous concentration, and does better in the swallowing when it's left more on its own.

Aside from the swallowing tips, we'd work on words, sentences, enunciating and some back-and-forth conversations to keep me practicing words, to help me slur less.

I like to say it was a help, but the help unfortunately does not last. It's the damn progression of symptoms that gets me! Every time I go for a new round of therapy, it is because I've worsened and I need to learn more tips and ways to do the simple tasks of life. I hate that when I finish my bulk of therapy "this time," it will not be my last. That seems to be the vicious cycle as this disease progresses. Learn and relearn. Learn, and relearn.

As a result of great advancements to understanding the cause of Friedreich's Ataxia, new treatments are now emerging. *Alleluia!* These treatments address the causes of FA such as gene mutation, frataxin production, iron sulfur clusters, and mitochondrial function. Several of these treatments are in clinical trials, which require patient participation and I find great importance in volunteering myself to enhance medical research in the clinical trial world.

Organizations like FARA (Friedreich's Ataxia Research Alliance) became my best friend when I needed every ounce of support I could find in order to pave the road to navigate a life with FA.

FARA is a non-profit that dedicates their donations to research and trials, grants, and holding different types of events. Their website houses many links to information on FA, as well as a database of members willing to help one learn about FA and the different ways to get involved with fundraising or signing up for the Friedreich's Ataxia registry—which allows willing participants to enroll in clinical trials and research. I find this organization to still be very helpful to me, as it updates my awareness with the upcoming and latest news around FA! I believe it also helps FAmilies (family members of diagnosed individuals) to better understand and cope, as well as guides others just needing some education.

A few years back, I volunteered myself to be an FA Ambassador. Ambassadors can have all sorts of different jobs and because I have a knack for writing, I helped with some blog posts.

I interviewed individuals with FA and introduced them on FARA's website. I also wrote about certain fundraising events, sharing the ins and outs of the event.

One in St. Louis I really enjoy is called 'Art & Soul;' it is an event where items have been donated for a silent auction. Many are paintings, or sculpted objects, as well as: sports gear, jerseys, pictures, collectibles, amazing seats to a ballgame—mostly to see the St. Louis teams—weekend getaways, booze, and more booze (that's St. Louis for you), restaurant certificates and the list goes on and on! There is usually a buffet for dinner, an open bar, live music and lots of socializing with other FAers (if they come), their FAmily, groups of FA supporters and event planners. I've really enjoyed the couple of times I've gone, but hopefully, with the Covid-19 pandemic, it is still all happening the way it did before.

An annual event that probably tops the cake is the FARA Energy Ball in Tampa, Florida. I've only had the opportunity to go to one, but I will happily go again if able. It is one of the highest fundraising events for FA that I know of. The gist of the party is a live auction. There're some silent auctions that happen too, but the big dollar amounts come from the live auction. When I went, I wore a nice dress, hair and make-up done up right, I ate a fancy white tablecloth dinner and pretended I had thousands of dollars to bid on timeshares and puppies. Not only are the items auctioned off valued far beyond the money in my wallet; the tickets to even attend are high up there. I totally get why they're pricey, but because of travel finances and the price tag of this event, I need time to save before another one.

I've also been to an event in Oklahoma that is called 'The Cure FA Soirée.' It's a benefit for FARA, ultimately raising funds through silent auctions and donations with wonderful performances of individuals singing and playing instruments, and a queue of speakers comprised of a mix of FA-diagnosed individuals, researchers, doctors, etc. who share updates about the disease and heartfelt real-life stories. It was also a great opportunity to meet new faces, FA or not, and be connected over the main goal of finding a cure [or treatment] for FA.

One of my favorite fundraising events I've had the pleasure to partake in for three consecutive years was the Slim's Journey Walk /Run. It was held in Warrenton, MO, about 45 miles west of St. Louis. This was my first event participation I'd taken part in for any type of FA fundraising. The first year I did it, I had my mom and two friends join and it was pretty cool to meet a few more people with FA, as well as their families and other supporters. The next two years, I expanded my team to Eli, family and friends and was so touched by the love and support I received!

With FA being so rare, it speaks volumes when there is an isolated event for the specific disease. It was a fundraiser that gathered money from those who signed up for the walk /run as well as donations from companies, families, and individuals. It was held at a church, but obviously the walk /run route was much longer than the parking lot, so the walkers /runners /strollers went through the streets, ending at the church, where church members were waiting with lots of yummy homemade treats and breakfast foods for all to indulge in after the race.

Slim's Journey started in 2012 after Julie & Jeff's son, Slim (his nickname) was diagnosed, in 2011, with Friedreich's Ataxia. After learning there was nothing they could do to stop this disease, it did not sit well with them.

"Therefore, we decided supporting FARA while honoring God was something we *could* do." —Julie

And BAM! They formed Slim's Journey Walk /Run, which totaled $150,000 raised for FARA. After seven years of hosting this event, they passed over the torch to another FAmily in Missouri that will hold a similar walk /run called 'FAmily Strides.'

There's other FA events and fundraisers across the globe, but I wanted to shed light on the ones I've been to and know firsthand. Check out www.curefa.org to read the details on my posts about these events. It's very nice to know there are people working tirelessly to put these events on, but it is even nicer to see their faces there.

It really does make me feel not-so-alone with my battling symptoms when I see other FAers there. Even if they're at a different stage of their prognosis, it is always a comforting feeling to know the support in the room is that of individuals fighting the same battle as you.

CHAPTER SIX

When the Battle Began

I t was definitely not easy to get used to my new norm. The challenges that came with the disease scared the hell out of me as I continued to progress. It wasn't just the physical factors, but the emotional ones as well. Struggles hit me at different times and in random scenarios. Sometimes a simple task, like making my bed, would royally frustrate me; I may be extra clumsy that day and going back and forth from one side of the bed to the other would soak up so much time and energy—and I still had a full day ahead of me.

In the beginning, it was all about the acceptance of having FA, and that was quite a battle. For many days after my diagnosis, I went about my business as usual. I went to work and school and hid what clumsiness I could when with friends, classmates, and coworkers. I would come home and pretend like I hadn't just heard the worst news of my life only days before. But those days turned into weeks that turned into months, and I never grew the courage to tell anyone. I figured by not telling anyone, no one would talk about it, and nothing related to what I had gone through would be real.

My parents ended up sharing it with our family, but other than that, I wasn't ready to spill the beans to anyone else. I was in denial big time. If I was careful enough, and conscious of what I was doing physically, I was able to keep it under wraps pretty well. It took a lot of effort; but then, I had been successful in keeping my diagnosis to myself and the family, even though I knew others noticed the occasional clumsy spells.

Little did I know that there would come the point when all of this would become supremely out of my control. I think it took me a good year, maybe even eighteen months, to realize it was best for me to come to terms and accept fully the fact that I had a genetic disease that would most likely, and eventually, lead me to a full-blown dependency.

Once I allowed myself to accept the disease—like really, truly accept it—I felt ready to tell my close friends. Even though I had made up my mind about telling them, I still didn't have it in me to tell my story in person. I couldn't muster up the courage to go through with it like that, so I decided to write them a message on Facebook Messenger. I started it with something along the lines of, "I have something to tell you…" then laying it all out there, explaining the best I could about FA and adding something to lighten the mood like, "Now you know that I am not always drunk when I stumble…."

While writing everything down, I was lifting so much stress off my shoulders; it felt so good not to hide behind closed doors any longer. I believe I ended my message to my friends by leaving it open-ended, for them to respond and ask whatever questions they might have. I think almost immediately, a lot of them called to talk to me about it. *No one* shied away. That alone granted me the perseverance to continue to talk about it and tell more of my friends. I studied up on FA as more questions were being asked. Soon, I realized how I was actually generating an (albeit small) awareness about this condition.

It was just a matter of time before my condition worsened and the challenges multiplied…. *Story of my life!* Literally. But then things became a bit more adventurous, once I found out that I was pregnant in October of 2011. *Surprise!* When I first found out, I had mixed emotions. I felt scared because this was my first pregnancy, and I wasn't exactly sure how my personal experience was going to go. I remember the thought flashing through my mind of, *Will I be doing it alone?* I was happy, too, knowing I could get pregnant (because some women can't) and felt—more than anything—overjoyed that I was going to get to raise a child that I got to call mine.

I knew my changing body could result in the FA progressing further, and that left a long road ahead, with a lot of unknowns. FA is genetic, meaning that there was the possibility of my child having it, like me. The thought of that was terrifying, and I certainly did not want my child to deal with this, too. Adding that on top of having just recently accepted my diagnosis fully; on top of experiencing quite the serendipitous pregnancy—and I was a little stress ball.

Fun Fact: My mom used to have this stone plaque on a little easel in the bathroom and I would read it all the time when washing my hands. It said: "Serendipity: an unexpected but very delightful discovery."

I have always thought of my child this way.

My child's father, Joey, did not know I had FA, so shortly after telling him that I was pregnant, I dropped the bomb of having a genetic disease. It certainly wasn't the most ideal conversation, but it needed to happen. The conversation went on for days with new and different questions, where each question led me to feel a little more and more self-conscious. Not what any expecting mother needs! Joey and I did not have a solid base for a relationship, so it was nerve wracking to witness the future father of my child taking in everything that I myself had just begun to accept. I just couldn't read where exactly he sat with all of this life-changing info, and we didn't have the developed intimacy to connect deeply over these new and unexpected challenges.

To phrase it lightly, before the serendipitous pregnancy, we'd enjoyed each other's company for about a month or two, but eventually decided to go our separate ways. We were no longer in contact at that point, and I figured that was that!

But *oh boy*, was I wrong.

One day weeks after our parting, I left work early, feeling sick and extremely exhausted. My friend texted to hang out, and I jokingly asked her to bring a pregnancy test with her on her way over.

I was not really that serious about it, because I had taken a pregnancy test just six days prior and it had come out to be negative. I had only gotten the hunch to take it again because I felt so incredibly different than usual and was late with my menstrual cycle. I felt like I was constantly having an out-of-body experience, as though I was looking at myself from the outside; it was so odd and even weirder trying to explain it to people. I went days without feeling *present*. I felt tired—like I had never been before. I was literally falling asleep while eating my lunch at work. It was not a good look!

But I really didn't think I could actually be pregnant. Not really. I had been out drinking the weekend before, because the Cardinals were in the World Series… a big deal for STL. I remember going to the first bar with some friends and trying to drink a beer, but it was taking forever. I couldn't even finish, dumping it out once it had turned warm. A friend of mine who often took advantage of an opportunity to turn low alcohol tolerance into a joke about being pregnant, instantly said, "Ohhh, you're pregnant!" But since I'd taken a test earlier that day that had read negative, I thought I was confident in replying with a "No way!" Thing is, I'm not even sure what had drawn me to take a test that day, either. Maybe it was my intuition?

Either way, I didn't feel like myself at all that night, so I called it an early night.

That following Monday, my work week started—I was a part-time teacher's assistant (TA) at a preschool at the time—and I could not shake how tired I was. I was still due to start 'aunt flow,' but since I had taken a test only days prior that was negative, I just figured, *any day now*….

That whole work week, it was a struggle for me to stay awake and it felt like 'cold' symptoms were stirring, too. Once Friday rolled around—still no 'aunt flow' anywhere in sight—I was like, *OK, what the hell is going on with me?!* I was usually pretty timely with that stuff, so I was starting to feel like something was definitely up. Feeling horrible, I left work early, my friend came over with the pregnancy test and sure enough: Positive. Positive. Positive. I took three to make sure, and all of them showed the "+" sign within seconds!

So, it's true: you can get a false negative *and* a positive just days apart!

CHAPTER SEVEN

The Reveal

You think about that moment when you find out you're pregnant and assess all of the different ways you could share the news with your child's father. Make it simple, or fancy? Tell him straight up, or surprise him? It is something precious and should be memorable.

Joey and I went back about a year prior to getting pregnant; but then, our relationship was strictly as friends for most of that time. We knew each other through mutual friends and obviously took our relationship to a more intimate level about a month or two prior to the pregnancy, though as you know, had fizzled out of that romance a couple weeks before I found out I was pregnant.

Joey didn't know I had FA partly because I didn't say anything about it, and mostly because he'd just never questioned me or seemed to notice that anything was off. Our relationship wasn't super deep, so I didn't want to share anything related to FA unless we were meant to blossom. As I was still coming to accept it myself, I definitely didn't want to share something so heavy if I didn't have to.

Since Joey didn't know, he didn't see me as disabled, and I liked that. I did, however, hold a little guilt inside myself that I wasn't upfront from the get-go, but since neither one of us were planning to become parents so quickly, I've since let that go. I like to believe in that corny, cliche saying: "Everything happens for a reason." And there is *so much purpose* for our having a child together.

Ephesians 1:11 reminds us that God's plan has a greater purpose than what we can see, "...for He chose us in advance, and He makes everything work out according to His plan."

Once I found out I was pregnant, after showing my friend Rachael the positive pregnancy test, I was overcome with the urge to let Joey know, too. I was all sorts of emotional. I was nervous, wanted to puke, and was sweating and shaking, but also happy. Knowing I was bringing new life into the world was something to be joyous about.

I had always envisioned crafting up a cute pregnancy reveal for my husband, so I definitely didn't know how to go about sharing this news in the midst of our unique dynamic. I ended up telling him without much of a plan, mostly because I just couldn't hold it in any longer.

One night, I somehow had been coerced into being his sober ride home. Pulling over to the side of the road to 'word vomit,' I said, "I'm pregnant."

So *this* was my big reveal! Joey seemed calmer than I would have expected, but I don't think he was in a place to fully comprehend the life-changing news I had just shared. To my absolute surprise, he blurted out, with a grin on his face, "Good, I'm glad! I want a baby!"

I'm sure it was all the alcohol talking because, to my dismay, the next day he told me he wasn't sure about the events from the night before and that everything was a bit blurry. Once I showed him, for certain, a positive pregnancy test, I think there was some shock that took a few days to settle. I was biting my tongue to share the next piece of news, about FA, until he could fully process that a baby was cookin', but just the same, felt I needed to have the conversation sooner rather than later. I really doubt there's a formal way to tell someone about a disease diagnosis, so I was just kind of winging it.

"I know I just shared huge news about us having a baby, but hey, by the way, I have a genetic disease…." I had a million things running through my head as I told him: *What will he think? What if he doesn't want anything to do with the baby? Can I do this on my own? What will happen if our kid has FA? How do I juggle my FA and a baby? What kind of relationship will Joey and I have? Do we try for something together? Do we stay separated? Can I financially do this?*

I wouldn't be surprised to know that most people's minds circulate with a million questions when they first find out they're expecting, so even aside from FA, I had the stress part of my pregnancy down pat! I knew I was going to stay on the path of motherhood regardless of Joey's decision, but I was hoping he'd be a part of this journey, too. His decision wasn't as quick as mine, but eventually he accepted and took on the role of preparing for fatherhood. I was thrilled that I would have a partner in all this; someone to share in the experience of raising a baby. Raising *our* baby.

Once FA was out on the table, the decision of whether Joey should be tested to see if he was a carrier of the FA gene was up for consideration. I didn't weigh heavier on either side, knowing versus not knowing, but we did decide, eventually, to have Joey tested. To have FA, you have to inherit the FA gene from both parents. We already knew that I would pass on the FA gene, since that is all I have to offer, as I have FA. But if Joey was not a carrier, there would be no risk that our child would have FA—they would just be a carrier. However, if Joey were a carrier, then our child would have a fifty percent chance of having FA.

A blood test is required to check if you are a carrier or not and somehow the lab ran his test wrong, and we didn't get a clear answer. Joey did not redo the test, as my Neurologist gave his two cents that not knowing would probably cause less worry. Just think, if we knew Joey was a carrier, that would mean we still wouldn't be certain if our child has FA because there is a 50/50 chance. Any time we saw our kid trip or fall (which most do anyway), we'd probably jump to the idea of FA and worry. He recommended we get our child tested if we ever had concerns with his balance in the future. We took that advice, and I am so glad we did.

I would've liked to work on a deeper relationship with Joey, but from the beginning, my focus was mostly on building a solid friendship while seeing if a romance would blossom organically. I don't believe we were ever on the same level in terms of commitment, though, and so it never stuck.

I do empathize with Joey and his experience with this, I really do… how different and difficult it must be for him to be wrapped up in FA over a short-term flit of a relationship, now bound to me as the other half of his child; bound to this whole world of FA. I would very much like having a kid with a full-time partner, but I would also like to *not* have FA. But of *course* I feel this way—and so I see this in Joey's eyes too. But the complexities of our lives are what create us. Are what burn our fears away and give us the strength to fight, sing and cry out in a passion for living. For surviving it all; for carrying on. And so, we do the best we can with our own complexities, Joey and me. And for our son, we work to set the clearest, most loving and best example we can.

It was complicated to the outside world, sure, but it was better than forcing a partnership. Neither one of us had been faced with this scenario before, so we didn't know what to expect or really what to do. *That* we were together on; that we shared. We had lots of trial and error ahead of us, and just rolling with the punches as they came seemed to be what was the best for us both.

We both wanted to be involved parents, so the desire to work on a future spark faded for me while we focused on finding a good groove and schedule in being as involved of parents as we could, separately.

Because I remained single throughout the whole pregnancy, I leaned on my parents and friends. I am very blessed to have many loved ones who've always supported me and spent quality time with me throughout the pregnancy. My favorite way to spend that quality time was going out to eat for breakfast. One of my biggest cravings included *all* breakfast foods. I could never make up my mind on a particular plate, so I would order à la carte: a chocolate chip Belgian waffle, cheesy hashbrowns, extra crispy bacon, biscuits and gravy, two fried eggs with buttered wheat toast and a side of maple syrup to dip my bacon into…. These items were my go-tos and it was always a little slice of heaven—in every bite!

And I kid you not: This one time, I had to push another table over to fit all these plates in front of me. I do not know how I didn't just blow up right there, but somehow, throughout my pregnancy, I either stayed right on track with my weight or was even underweight. Now all I do is look at a piece of bread and gain five pounds. *Why?!?* I miss that metabolism! Fortunately though, besides fatigue and nausea, I didn't experience many other major pregnancy symptoms. However, I soon learned that dealing with FA and pregnancy would present me with other challenges.

Right at the end of my first trimester, I had a fall that freaked me out so badly that I rushed to the E.R. My balance was progressively getting worse, which my doctor had told me could happen more readily while pregnant. I slipped on the bottom of my sweatpants, which had wrapped under the bottom of my heels, and without the ability to catch myself, fell directly onto my belly. Just typing this out makes me feel so silly—that I was so *careless*!

I was so scared of the thought that something terrible had happened to the baby, that I had my mom come over, and we went right to the hospital. I was in hysterical mode and couldn't relax at all until I heard the baby's heartbeat on the monitor. Thankfully, the baby was fine; however, I was not. This incident was the sign to start using an assistive device. I dreaded this realization, but I needed to protect myself in order to protect this little human in my belly!

During that time, I had read about this study that was conducted between thirty-one pregnant women with FA, where information about their medical history, history of pregnancy and delivery, and feelings about pregnancy related to having FA were all collected[7]. Interestingly, there were mixed results when it came to this last question. Eight women believed that pregnancy improved their FA symptoms (most saying their coordination and balance had improved); ten women felt their symptoms had gotten worse (most saying that fatigue had increased, followed by urinary urgency and then an increase in speech, balance, and coordination issues); and thirteen did not feel that pregnancy affected their FA at all. Literally, pregnancy with FA could go in any direction.

Again, yet another big unknown! However, I was accepting the fact that my balance and coordination *were* declining more quickly and that I needed to be safe about this. It wasn't just about me anymore.

This was when I began that first journey of physical therapy and found my walker. Remember *Sylvia*? McKenzie, my physical

---

[7] Friedman, Lisa S. "Pregnancy with Friedreich Ataxia: a Retrospective Review of Medical Risks and Psychosocial Implications." AJOG, 17 May 2019, www.ajog.org/article/S0002-9378(10)00365-0/fulltext.

therapist, was pregnant too and we were due just days apart, so we quickly bonded over being on the same timeline of pregnancy. I feel she also became a bit of a barometer for me, in terms of what my pregnancy would look like without FA, so I could see the contrast in our journeys and know firsthand what was and was not "normal." My sessions of exercise and learning new tasks sometimes became talks about babies, which made it all the less stressful and scary for me.

As my hands were always occupied holding the walker, I couldn't hold onto things while walking, which was especially annoying for me while being pregnant! Bumps and cracks in the streets sucked. Cooking was harder. Bringing my plate of food to the table felt nearly impossible. I had to rely on water bottles, as there were bound to be puddles of water on the ground if I tried to carry a cup. Everything took longer, with more concentration and awareness. I could no longer just "slip my shoes on," or "hop in the shower," or "run an errand really quick." I could only get dressed and undressed from a seated position. I now had to sit on a shower chair in order to shower in the tub. Getting into and out of the car and stabilizing myself took more effort than I wanted. I needed to make sure I grabbed a shopping cart to walk with at the store, even if I was picking up two items. I wasn't able to look down and see my feet while walking with the big belly, which didn't help my focus while walking. I felt the weight of the baby, my back hurt, and sleeping just wasn't comfortable.

As more trials went on, I was finding my groove, even though some tasks had me wanting to lay in the fetal position and just cry my eyes out. But I sucked it up until it got easier. I lived alone, so I felt that I had no choice but to learn, for example, how to bring my dirty clothes to the wash machine to do my laundry with the limitations that I had. Looking back, I am in awe of the strides I was able to take in navigating FA and pregnancy all alone. I learned and relearned so much in terms of my capabilities. I give that trial-and-error period of my life so much credit to my independence today. Since then, I appreciate assistance, but I do like to accomplish as much as I can independently, or at least try things myself before asking for help.

On January 19th, 2012, Joey and I went to see the doctor and found out we were having a boy! We were so excited and couldn't wait to tell our parents. We wanted to do something easy and creative (this was before gender reveals were so popular), so we bought a couple of balloons that said, "It's A Boy," wrapped them in trash bags (super classy) and gave one to each of our parents. We then watched them open them up, the balloons floating to the ceiling as their excitement grew. Those were very memorable moments and I still smile whenever I think about them!

As days and weeks went by, we got accustomed to getting all the boyish things bought and ready for our little guy's arrival. I loved shopping a bit more than I usually would! It turns out it is *so* hard to say "no" to the cute little shoes that no newborn really even needs. It's not like he is going to be walking himself to the car, but how do I turn down baby-sized converse?! This could be the most important $35 I'd ever spend!

CHAPTER EIGHT

My Kiddo

June 10th, 2012, at 12:44 am, weighing 7 pounds, 8 ounces, and measuring 21 inches long, Elijah 'Eli' Joseph graced us with his presence on his exact due date! He was beyond perfect. The moment I saw my child for the first time, feeling his skin, watching his chest move up and down, and hearing his tiny little cry, gave me all the feels. It was pure joy. An indescribable love only other parents would likely understand.

I went into the hospital on June 7th to be induced, thinking Eli would be here the next day, June 8th. *Ehhh…* not so much.

It took a lot to get Eli here.

Because of FA, there were concerns of an epidural, as there was the chance of permanent nerve damage /paralysis. *Everyone* is at a small risk for that happening, but as I already have a disease that affects my nerves, it was a risk I really had to consider.

When you get a C-Section and are awake, you either have an epidural or spinal block; so, risky business if I went that route, too. The docs talked about the possibility of knocking me out and having a C-Section that way, so I would only need local anesthesia instead of an epidural or spinal block, but I was super upset about the potential of not being awake for Eli's delivery; plus I really wanted to have a natural birth.

I did two rounds of induction (Cervidil and Pitocin twice). After my second round, I was only dilated 2cm. You need to be at 10cm to deliver, though, so I had a long way to go. It was now June 9th, and the slow process was draining me. Two days of being in the hospital, trying to get the ball rolling, and I was at a whopping 2cm! *Are you kidding me?!*

My doctor encouraged me to just go home and let nature run its course, but being there for forty-eight hours really brought out the brand new mama bear in me: "I'm not leaving here without my baby!" I demanded.

My doctor was okay with my decision, but she did recommend that I allow her to break my water to speed things up. This decision could result in a C-Section if the waiting game took too long, but at this point, I was like, "Sign me up!"

Minutes after my water broke, my contractions came with full force. I swear, labor is probably the worst pain I've ever encountered. I do not tolerate pain well, so it didn't take long before I was puking from the intense contractions. The nurse saw how much pain I was in and kept pushing me to get an epidural, but I was trying to keep myself amped up for doing this completely naturally, and so was the doula I had hired to assist my delivery. For those who don't know, a doula is someone who provides guidance and support while a pregnant woman is in labor. I stayed strong for a couple of hours, but eventually, I did give in to the epidural. Even with the risks, I had to ease the pain, and it was the best decision I could've made. That stuff is like liquid gold! Seriously.

I was pain-free for the remaining few hours, but I'll never forget how I was only numb on one side. I could move my left leg and wiggle my toes, but the whole right side was like a dead weight. I also had the most intense shivers; I couldn't stop from feeling like I was outside in the middle of winter, slowly dying from the cold. I found out that this was a side effect of the epidural, but I just couldn't stop clattering my teeth. Truthfully, though, I'd take that over the labor pains any day!

To this day, I don't really know what happened in those final moments before pushing. Lots of medical professionals in the room, discussing something as they moved me over to one side and started pushing on my belly to move the baby…. I think the baby's heart rate dropped. Or was he in distress? I don't know. I'm glad I was never told, to be honest. After the nurses were satisfied with my dilation, they said it was time, and that the doctor would be coming in shortly. That's when it all became *so* real!

I am extremely grateful that I didn't have to push more than thirty minutes before my baby was here. It was an intense three days, but so worth it all! It's true what they say: "The pain goes away as soon as you hold your baby." Maybe it was the epidural still numbing me out, or adrenaline and pure joy surging through me, but I surely felt perfect holding my baby.

Coming home from the hospital then opened up a whole new can of "mommy worries" and "what-ifs." Even though I had learned a great deal about taking care of myself months prior, I now needed to do it for a tiny human who only knew how to sleep, breathe, eat and cry—as well as provide huge blowouts in his diapers! Joey stayed at my house the first few weeks, but after that, I was on my own. I had visitors and went over to my parents' at times, but I needed and wanted to learn what I should as a single mom. I felt I needed to own my new responsibilities.

Besides my Super Mom powers, I learned a great deal of different techniques in taking care of myself and a baby at the same time.

When Eli was a newborn, up until he started walking, I was able to take care of him by myself at my house. I put him in a bassinet on wheels or a stroller to move him around the house. He slept next to my bed in a pack n' play. I had his bottles all set up on my nightstand, so I was always ready for those late night, middle of the night, and early morning feedings. Was it difficult?

Hell yea! Was I exhausted? More than ever! But I wouldn't have felt like a new mom if I hadn't experienced that on my own.

I did get frustrated; especially at the little things: dropping Eli's binky on the floor, spilling his formula all over, cleaning up all his toys, washing the endless pile of dirty clothes or the *worst*, when Eli would be crying, and I could only sit to hold him. Like most babies, Eli loved to be held while standing, but I couldn't do it. I hated that I couldn't. I beat myself up for it.

The extreme exhaustion was a new level of tiredness. There were many times I fell asleep in the middle of feeding Eli a bottle or gave him extra milk so that he would soothe himself to sleep and I could get that extra hour of sleep myself. Mom struggles!

I just get tickled pink whenever I hear that classic nugget of wisdom everyone wants to share with a new mom: "Sleep when the baby sleeps!" Great, sensible advice. Absolutely!

Also: *impossible*.

During the day, I'd have tons of things to get done that could only happen when Eli was asleep. There was no way I could shut my brain off to rest due to the heavy amounts of caffeine I had already pumped through my body to function for the earlier part of my day, so I figured I may as well down some more caffeine to start prepping for the latter part. Once I was "jacked up on Mountain Dew," I would really just want to sit and watch my perfect baby sleep, dream, and make his widdle baby noises.

After staring unblinkingly at a sleeping Eli through most of his nap, admiring his beautiful features, I would be left with only about forty-five minutes to accomplish the following: do some laundry, clean the dishes, eat something besides a bag of chips, take a glorious hot shower, and maybe, just maybe, reply to a text message that had been awaiting my response. There's absolutely no way I was ever able to do all these things, though, so I would have to consider which was the most important at that time: *What's one more day without a shower? I'll just keep re-fluffing the clothes in the dryer and pulling items to wear until I've worn everything*—my motto to this day! *I'll keep using dishes from the clean dishwasher until it's ready to run again. I'll just open another box of Cheez-its, I'll respond to everyone on my phone during Eli's next nap, and once I get a good night's sleep, I can knock it all out tomorrow.* Ha! Ha! Triumph!

All jokes aside, I still wonder how the hell I did it. I personally think I morphed into this person that just kept going and going. I haven't stopped and I don't think that ever goes away, once you become a parent. I haven't had a good night's rest since 2011.

And sure, I can cry, complain, and scream all I want in my most overwhelming of moments, but the big girl pants have to come back on after a meltdown. *They* say, "You'll grow up fast when you have a kid," and my goodness, they aren't kidding.

I was and still am proud of the work and creativeness I put toward being as independent as I could be at the time. I learned a lot from it, and as much as I wish I could remember every hack I'd come up with—because let's face it, I hardly remembered to make myself a nutritious hot meal most days—I pretty much nailed it with Eli, as a baby and as a toddler!

As time progressed, Eli became more mobile and active, which in turn made it very challenging to stop him from climbing all over the place—to the point where I'd spend most of my days just chasing him down. I don't know about you, but the mischievous attitude and always-running pitter patter of a newly walking baby is frustrating beyond words. Cute, adorable—but frustrating. "No," "Get down," "Stop," and "You'll get hurt," were my new [not so] favorite vocabulary words that I got more than annoyed at hearing myself say. Because of these inevitable, temporary, and difficult changes, my parents opened their doors for us to stay with them for a while. I still enjoyed the independence I had at my own home, though, so I eventually got into the rhythm of staying with my parents when I had Eli and taking advantage of being at my house for freedom whenever Eli was with Joey. We had a mutual split custody agreement, which gave Eli the time to soak up both parents, equally and separately.

I will always be extremely grateful to my parents for helping and being there for us. Just because my parents were around didn't mean everything was easy-peasy, though! I may have needed help with bathing Eli, cooking meals, and chasing him down, but I'm still his mom: I played with him, we ate our meals together, I changed his diapers, got him dressed, drove him around, disciplined him, cuddled with him, read to him, and we would watch movies together.

There was still a line between grandparents and parents, and I feel we had it down pretty well.

We kept that cycle going until Eli was almost five. The house I called "mine" was a home I rented from my aunt and uncle. It was a small slab home that had been in the family for years. It had been my great grandparents' home many moons ago, then my cousins', then my aunt and uncle had bought it, which allowed me to then rent it from them. After the wonderful time I'd spent in that home, my aunt and uncle were planning to sell it, and since I was in no position to purchase at the time, I moved into my parents' house full time. It was a bit saddening to leave that independent part of my life behind. I am an adult mother and didn't want to have the label of "living with mommy and daddy," no matter what my life circumstances were.

I was able to acclimate to my new living arrangement and realized how having my parents close by was beneficial and how it was much more of a blessing than any sort of frustration, to have their support and assistance when needed.

Eli has also learned, over the years, my dos and don'ts, and has become a very generous helper. Once he grew to be more comprehensive, Eli was able to carry things for me or do a simple task here and there to help me out. I tried and still do try not to ask for too much, so that he doesn't feel like I'm relying on him. He's a kid and I'm the parent, so I don't dump any adult responsibility on him. I do, at times, struggle with the balance of what I should and shouldn't ask, but I write that off as it is something that comes with the territory of parenting and is a unique challenge to discern through in our situation.

Now over nine years old, he is independently capable of doing much more, negating the need for me to feel like I'm burdening him; plus, some things are just great life lessons for him, and he approaches them like a gentleman. These include bringing groceries or bags in from the car, pouring glasses of water for dinner, cleaning up after himself, carrying my plate of food to the table, holding open the door, carrying something up or down the stairs for me, making smoothies (his favorite), and he just knows what to do without me even asking, at this point. He's only known me since I've been using an assisted device; so to him, it's second nature to chime in and help me out when needed.

I'm so proud. And on top of it all, Eli is a very handsome boy! I know, I know… I'm partial! But I swear he is. He has brown eyes and brown hair. A great complexion—he tans so well! He looks a lot like his dad, I think, but the older he gets, people say he's looking more and more like me. He's of average height for his age, but he looks like he'll be a tallish man. He's got a small waist, but strong arms and legs. Sports seem to come naturally to him. He doesn't necessarily enjoy playing all sports, but he's got the athletic knack for it when he wants to.

And he is *so* smart! When he was only two years old, I bought him a placemat to put under his plates of food that had all the U.S. presidents on it. He would study it every time he ate and by the time he was four years old, he knew the order and name of every president! The family was in awe of his reception! I still am. I only know like five presidents!

During our car rides, Eli loves for me to quiz him on certain things he's taking an interest in at the time. Right now, it's all the state capitals and he, of course, knows them all! He's refreshed my mind as I am relearning them. We've also done quizzes about all the baseball and hockey teams, and the players on our city's team. One time, it was all about the makes and models of different cars. He's a walking encyclopedia!

He also loves naming the cities and states he'd like to live in when he's older. So far, it's been: Colorado, California, Alabama, Oregon, Savannah, Georgia, and currently, it is Chattanooga, TN. I'm excited to hear what's next on his list.

Being in my condition, I am still able to provide for Eli, which I am extremely grateful for. He goes to school in Joey's district, which is about a twenty-five-minute drive for me, so being able-bodied enough to drive is something I do not take for granted. Driving to and from school are great times for us to chat and play "I spy…" or other car games. I also drive Eli to his sporting and school events on the days he's with me. Many play dates are with friends from school; so, again, I occasionally take part in the pickup or drop off. I am so used to the drive by now, it's a route

I can do with my eyes closed. Don't fret, though—I'll be sure to keep these eyes on the road!

I am afraid that there *are* real struggles Eli does face as a result of my life with FA. Since I must take side roads whenever I drive, it's typically a longer route and like most kids, twenty minutes feels like hours, so Eli does get frustrated and becomes very vocal about how much "FA sucks" because I can't drive on highways to get to places more quickly. When we go to the store or out to eat, just us two, he will also get frustrated that it takes me longer to get out of the car and wheel myself around. Or a little embarrassed when people stare.

It doesn't bother me, but to a kid, having stares really does embarrass him.

Once, when Eli and I went with some family to the Wisconsin State Fair, he refused with tears of anger that he wouldn't go down the slide without me. My cousin Elise had just gone down with her daughter, so Eli was probably thinking, *What about me and my mom?*

Because of my lack of coordination and the need to stabilize my trunk, it wasn't practical or safe for me to go down this high of a slide, with as many dips as it had. I told Eli I wasn't going to do it, but that Elise or her husband, David, would go with him instead. He was not having that. He cried and stumped on the ground and said, "I hate FA!"

I was sad I couldn't go down the slide with him that day, and cursed FA for taking that memory away from us, and for taking that experience away from him.

Thus, I try to be as independent as I can be, where it comes to Eli. When we take airplane trips, just us two, from time to time, he walks by my side as I am pushed by a skycap through the airport. He's very well behaved during our flights and listens to all my instructions to remain safe.

Traveling can be tough for any age and capability; I pat myself on the back for navigating it with my kid all on our own! It's a big achievement, I think, and I believe we can continue to travel together as time moves forward—plus, with Eli getting older, that means more maturity and independence on his part, so it may only get easier for us.

Over the years, parenthood changes. My worries aren't making sure Eli isn't putting his finger in the outlet or eating Cheerios he finds in between the couch cushions anymore; it's making sure he does his homework, explaining how money doesn't grow on trees, teaching chores and responsibilities, talking about friendships and being loyal, listening and giving advice about his sadness rather than just kissing a 'booboo' to make everything better, and the best of all: just loving him dearly—while saying *WTF!* to myself several times a day! I wish it were still as easy as sleep, eat, potty, repeat, but he's getting older and wiser; Eli's need for *Mom* will always be there, though the necessity of it changes. Eli makes me so proud, and I am in constant awe of his kindness and generosity. I can't take credit for all of it, but knowing he is absorbing some of the life lessons I've instilled makes my heart feel warm and fuzzy. I feel grateful and at peace.

I can't compare what it'd be like having a togetherness with Joey as a parent versus not, as we've been separated since Eli was born—even so far back as to when he was but a bun in the oven— so I really have no idea what it could've been like if, at any point, we'd taken the alternate path. There are times where I've imagined what it could be like, but I bet my visions are pretty farfetched from the truth, so I don't really beg them to linger.

When I would get very frustrated or doubtful as a mother, or learned that I'd missed out on witnessing some amazing "first" life event of Eli's because he was with Joey at the time, I'd get upset and come to the conclusion that these things wouldn't happen if Joey and I were partners. I'm sure he's missed out on many firsts due to this same thing, as well. But I would think of how great it'd be if we were doing this together, as a loving, close-knit-bond couple, raising our kid together.

In some ways this vision was only due to feeling perturbed in the moment, though, as I would quickly thereafter change my tune and find peace and appreciation for having jumped the many hurdles and endured the many hardships I have from doing so much on my own with Eli.

I've made it this far and so has Eli; over nine years later and he is *crushing* it as a kid! Honestly, to say I'm proud is an absolute understatement. I don't have the words for how much I love him, how proud I am of him, and how honored I am to be his mama.

CHAPTER NINE

Friends, Family, and Colleagues

As the clocked ticked on, I witnessed as FA became more and more normalized in my circle. There were still questions asked, but I didn't experience the same shyness in answering them. My disease was becoming more accepted and feeling more normal for me to address head-on.

I don't believe that Friedreich's Ataxia really *changed* me—or so that is what I like to think. If anything, it brought more confidence out from within me. More openness, transparency, and will to do what I needed to do to live the life I desired. I feel like I still have a lot of the same interests as I'd had before the diagnosis. I am a social person and like to go out and about with my friends and do kid-stuff with Eli. I do not know what it's like to be short on friendships; I feel very blessed to have many. A large chunk of my friends are from high school, some even as far back as grade school, so we're pretty tight-knit; plus it *is* St. Louis—everyone is connected in some way, shape or form.

During college and just after undergrad, my friends and I were still living the "let's go to the bar on a Tuesday" life, while throwing in just a few of the responsibilities of young adulthood. Some of us were moving out of our parents' homes to find places of our own, others finding the career they've been searching and interviewing for, and some even continuing in education with bigger goals and dreams in mind.

Just after college, I was planning to work at a preschool with the goal to pursue grad school and work in counseling, but I wanted to soak up my newfound freedom first, as I was experiencing the feeling of relief in no longer needing to lock myself in with a pile of books to study. Plus, I knew that once it was time to knuckle back into it, I would need to allow my diagnosis to take the front seat so that I could move forward with how it would play into my life goals regarding school, work and a family… in the future.

But, once I was pregnant, and then had a kid, my timeline of goals really shifted and many of my dreams had to be fast-tracked. I'd gotten pregnant only ten months after finishing undergrad, so with throwing FA into the mix, I had to push the pause button on a few of the things I'd been aiming for. I also had given birth years before the majority of my friends were starting down that road, so there have been times since where we really aren't in harmony as a result. Not in a negative way, just that our responsibilities were and still are a bit different from one another's. Plus, I was trying to adapt to a life with an altering disease. FA and a baby were clearly asking to be my main focus.

Since the beginning, I don't feel like any of my friends have ever shunned me away because of my FA. I have always found them to be very supportive and empathetic towards my needs. I've even had two fundraisers put together by friends and family. *That right there* is love. We still do all the things friends do: brunch, dinners, movies, weddings, baby showers, birthday parties, random get togethers, and such, but as I've gotten older and my kid is now past the toddler stage, they are just starting to get married, have kids and form their own families.

Even though my life looks totally different from theirs, I am so happy for them. They are in a different phase of life, so maybe we see each other less, but they're my besties, 'til death do us part. Some friends are going on double dates; others are organizing play dates for their group of kids; some experience the sleepless nights of raising their first kid or even multiple children, while others are busy with career progression, the responsibilities of being a homeowner, etc. There has been a time or two where I've fallen into the sadness of missing the times when we could meet up and hang at the drop of a hat, but adulting is hard work, even taking FA out of the equation.

I experience constant reminders that even though life isn't remotely close to what I'd envisioned, adapting to what life gives us is the secret to happiness.

Now that Eli is getting older and forming friendships of his own, I've also started to become friends with some of his friends' parents. It's very nice having that common groove of our kids to connect over. We enjoy playdates, lunch dates, sports activities and all the things boys like to do with their friends, all while we moms sit to "chitchat," as Eli likes to say. Plus, being able to escape on our own for some drinks and conversations that aren't interrupted every two minutes has a feeling of its own. A feeling of some much-needed R&R. Adult conversations. Adult beverages.

Being the only child on my side, Eli has developed close bonds with many of his cousins, which is exactly what I had done growing up, and it warms my heart knowing (and hoping) that he'll still have those close relationships as he gets older. Technically, they're my cousins' kids, which makes them like his second cousins or something, but their bond is close, so we just say "cousins," and I hope that they will be the ones to keep the family traditions alive when the older generations are no longer able.

I've also made some friends who have my condition, but they don't live in St. Louis. I know only about five people who have FA around the STL area. The out-of-towners I have befriended are because of FARA and different groups that, fortunately, have connected us. Because FA is rare, social media and online support groups are the biggest way for us all to connect. The groups are a great platform for us to ask questions related to FA, or to posit any other life struggles to others with FA or FAmily who can offer their two cents. It has brought many together, in getting the opportunity to learn so much more of how FA impacts people differently, and to give us all the sense of 'not being alone.'

These groups and the friends I've made through them have also allowed me to be invited to visit them in their various cities. As well, I've had the pleasure to meet face-to-face with most of the people I've met through research trials and fundraising events.

The very first person I ever met who had FA, I connected with while taking part in a research trial in Tampa, FL. She lives in Michigan, and even though neither one of us ever visited the other in our hometowns, we were able to get to know one another through our many visits to Tampa for the same trial that we were taking part in; plus, through our communication via social media and texts sent back and forth, we really got to know one another after a while. She has since passed away from cancer and I commemorate her for her strength in navigating two very life-altering diagnoses like that. I miss her positive energy and think of her often. I will see her again one day, but until then, kicking FA in the ass is what I'll keep doing!

I've been to Atlanta, Oklahoma, and Tampa to visit with friends and attend events (as well as some in my home state, too). With my many visits to Florida for research trials, meeting others who have FA has become a bit of a domino effect over the years. I would also end up forming relationships with all of their FAmily, so my circle has really grown over the years, thanks to the strands that connect those of us who have been affected by FA. I sure am humbled to know and love so many groups of people; you can never have too many beautiful people in your life.

It is pretty easy to be around people who have a similar condition to mine. I was standoffish in meeting someone with FA for many years because I was afraid I'd lose that sense of "normalcy." I just didn't want to be defined by FA and I was nervous that I wouldn't like seeing a mirror image of myself. Of course, I was wrong. When I allowed myself to welcome the community of FA, we could all relate to and understand one another's trials, mishaps, and appreciations. There's a special connection in being around others who travel along the same road as you. I love meeting all ages and prognoses of FA! All their stories were and still are enlightening. I've learned so much.

However, there is the downside to being around those who portray tons of negative energy—really whether they have FA or not. I am more of an optimistic person, so that pessimism can be draining for me to be around. I try to be sensitive to those who are down in the dumps, because they may have it a lot harder than me, and it does indeed get sad and depressing. I also like to think that no matter what you go through, each person should take as much time as they need to sulk about it, grieve, etc.; but also, you shouldn't stay in the 'sulking' state of mind forever, as you'll end up missing out on the goodness of the life you *do* have yet to lead.

For me, it is always hard to see people suffering, especially when it is from FA. I end up going down a rabbit hole in my mind when I see someone who is really struggling with their symptoms because I get super nervous about developing symptoms similar to what I witness. And I think that's another reason why I don't judge the thought that arises in me, of "this could be me in five years." I'd prefer to think, "No, I won't be a Negative Nancy," but you never really know; our lives are made of change. I've had to learn to accept change when it comes. And just because I don't have a negative mentality now, doesn't mean I couldn't develop it due to my worsening condition or surrounding situations.

I can't think about that too much or I start getting anxious over something that isn't even there, though! I just hope that I stay the same with the positive attitude I have cultivated. It really keeps me afloat and, I believe, keeps me doing as well as I am. Having a positive attitude while dealing with this condition takes a lot; but then, it allows me to aspire and to hope. It allows me to grow. With a positive mentality, you're more apt to allow people into your life who accept you for you, help you, and love you despite whatever it is you're going through.

I've allowed myself to be vulnerable and accept so much love and friendship in my life because I choose to find the good. I do have days where I want to sulk and feel sorry for myself, which sometimes is totally necessary and actually healthy—to let out the frustration—but I know that I'll probably face a pretty shitty outlook that whole day afterwards, as a result of setting that sort of negative mindset as the foundation for my day. I just feel like I'm extra clumsy and cannot complete my tasks in a timely manner whenever I do get into a negative mindset.

On those days, it takes a real self-pep-talk to get back into the flow of positivity. It's hard, but very much needed for me to keep from being knocked down by FA. FA is strong as shit! It sometimes feels like a wave that wants to crash over me, and I just need to keep surfing, laser focused all the way through. All it takes is one little FA mishap, and I can quickly slip into being a Debbie Downer, lose my focus, and have a terrible time... so I choose to find the good, and embrace the changes with grace when I can.

CHAPTER TEN

Dating

ERIN K PIEPER

Pregnancy and the acceptance of my FA did not occur far apart from each other, so my number one priority for a while was just accepting and learning as much as I could about the two things together. As a result, I really didn't start dating again until years after Eli was born. I was a little nervous about how a potential partner could view my disability, especially alongside my already being a mom. Not just anyone could understand what my condition was due to the rarity of it, so dating a woman with a disability *and* a kid is a door not many are willing to walk through.

Dating is hard enough for an able-bodied person; throw in a wheelchair and it goes from difficult to almost not worth the trouble. I know I possess many of the things most people desire when searching for a partner—I just so happen to do activities mostly from a seated position. If I could, I would send this wheelchair packing, but I need my wheels; they're my legs.

For better or worse, my wheelchair sets me apart. But in dating? It's mostly worse.

I find that most of the resistance to dating someone in a wheelchair is due to the stigma that wheelchair users are dependent and weak and poor and sad and sick and can't perform in the bedroom, and so much more… but I am here, of course, to spread the knowledge and awareness that people who use a wheelchair to maneuver around aren't always those things and may not even align with a single one of them. I can't speak for every wheelchair user and say we're all "datable" and "spouse material," because, frankly, that isn't true either; however, I bet many wheelchair users are. We're just not given the chance to show how great we are when someone *only* sees the wheels.

Would you treat me differently if you didn't see the wheelchair or walker? I'd like a man to just simply treat me like a woman. Be interested, if interested, instead of allowing FA to be the dealbreaker. Court me. Send me flowers. I'd like to be dated and liked just like any able-bodied woman.

I think most people wouldn't see me as so "not normal" if the world didn't already implant the view of disabilities as pitiful. I roll my eyes when, at first, I hear all the compliments from a guy, like, "you're pretty, beautiful, gorgeous…" or, "you're sweet, kind, and have a wonderful personality…" and then, once they learn about the wheelchair, I'm met with crickets. Pregnant pauses. Dumbfounded, pained expressions. It's frustrating and just plain annoying. There needs to be a huge societal pivot, where we stop shoveling all this fear between wheelchairs and love. Where we leave some space to learn more about the individual before rejecting the idea of dating altogether.

I see so many people who are in a relationship with a significant other who has a mental illness, a drug addiction, obesity, abuse, controlling behaviors, cancer, a life altering disease or just unhealthy dynamics, so why does it seem that wheelchair users, specifically, have a harder time being in a partnership? Why is *an assistive device* the hard stop? I ask myself this question quite often and try to answer from what I hear, read, watch or from personal experiences. I've gathered that, perhaps, it could be because:

- We're seen to potentially implode a relationship, as we are often "too much" to handle, financially, physically, and emotionally.
- People worry they're going to have to take on the role of "caregiver."
- They think they will have to shift all their hobbies to be more "handicap-friendly."
- They take it upon themselves—before even being intimate—to presume that intimacy will be awkward, frustrating, or scarce.
- They are intimidated by the potential challenges that may come along over time.

- Society may judge, or make fun. Or someone close to them won't be supportive.
- They think you already have a death sentence set.

These may come across as believable or even acceptable reasons to you because, well, civilization has probably already embedded them into your head—but they're all assumptions. You truly don't know whether any of these things are true unless you take the time to get to know the particular wheelchair user from the inside.

Before I get into my own dating journey, allow me to share a particular situation that happened a while back with my own wheelchair that proves just how wrong assumptions can be:

One time, when I went to a local baseball game with a group of friends, we did not have seats in an accessible section, so I, in my carefree way, hitched a ride on a friend's back to get down the stairs to our seats. I asked the usher who was patrolling that section where I could leave my wheelchair and he reassured me he'd be close by, and to just fold it up and lean it against the wall by the stairs so it would be under his radar.

Done.

After a few innings, I had to go to the restroom and got piggy backed back up to the main level. Once we got up there, I looked left, looked right, but there was no sign of my wheelchair or the usher. Once I got plopped down somewhere to sit, we started looking around and within five minutes, the usher came waltzing back. I asked him, "Why isn't my wheelchair here?" and he instantly responded in panic mode, "I've been on break for thirty minutes. It was here when I left!"

I said, "Oh no, this isn't good!" But I thought, *WTF, dude! You said you'd be able to keep an eye on it for me!*

After getting more people involved in the hunt for the wheelchair, the head honchos were called, and the stadium was put on lockdown. Some serious shit. No one could leave the stadium without being checked out first—but let's face it… it's a wheelchair. You can't really miss it.

Anyway, enough time had passed to where we realized that, if it was stolen, the thief was long gone and out of those doors already. The clock was ticking, and I felt so helpless. I mean, that wheelchair is practically my legs. My mobility. My independence.

Once the game ended, I was in the same boat of having no wheelchair and the stadium employees gave me an "apology gift" and a golf cart ride out to the car. I said to them, "Thank you, but what am I supposed to do when I get home? I don't have my wheelchair!" All they could say in return was, "I'm sorry and we'll have more answers for you tomorrow."

Ummmmm, ok?!?!

Luckily, I did have a very crappy, hand-me-down wheelchair at home to use in the meantime. However, the wheelchair topper I use in my car is designed only to work with my MIA wheelchair, so that made things even more frustrating. I felt so many mixed emotions, of being sad, mad, frustrated, embarrassed, dependent….

I made sure to file a stolen property report with St. Louis PD that night, and the next day, after many back-and-forth phone calls with the baseball organization, the only news I got was, "We're working on it. Our team is having a meeting today on what we can do for you."

That turned into seven days of, "We're looking into it." Can you imagine going seven days with no legs and no one to direct you in how to cope with that?!

It was tough. But life still was happening. There was no pause button. My kid still needed to go to and from school. I still had to find a way to get to my scheduled appointments. I still had to attend and get around for my work events. I had to have friends throw my "not so good" wheelchair in the trunk and help me in and out of the car.

It sucked, to say the least.

More back and forth phone calls until *finally* they got something. A coordinator from the organization sent me info on the guy who had stolen my wheelchair and was now selling it on Facebook Marketplace. I almost threw up. I couldn't believe I was looking at my wheelchair that this person had stolen right out of the park!

With my amazing Facebook skills, I tracked down this guy pretty quickly and contacted the Granite City, IL police department about his attempt to sell my property. Two officers went to his house; he was not home, but his dad was, and freely let the officers into the home to take my wheelchair. Once I received that phone call, I was so beyond relieved.

I went to Illinois to retrieve my wheels, but if I wanted to press charges, it looked like it was going to be sticky. The crime happened in St. Louis, MO and they took it over state lines to sell it in Illinois. So I needed the St. Louis police department to hand the crime over to Granite City, but that meant I couldn't take it, in case they needed to run it for prints. I tried for a couple of days to follow this path, but after not receiving any return calls, I decided to opt out of pressing charges so that I could actually use my wheels again. I left the whole thing thinking, "Just be thankful you got it back in one piece. Karma will get that guy. I've got my independence back!"

After what felt like the longest week ever, I was reunited with my independence.

This wheelchair *is* my legs; how would you feel if someone took your 'actual' legs, and you were left to figure out your every move without them?! Scared? Upset? Angry? Helpless? Dependent? All the above. It's shitty that I actually have to have a checklist stored in my head on how to navigate when my "legs" are stolen, should that ever happen again. Or if the wheelchair breaks. Or needs maintenance. No matter what kind of "legs" one has, they're absolutely essential for survival!

I was blessed with this customized wheelchair from vocational rehab—I still use it—and let me tell you… these aren't cheap. It's hard to be understanding when you find out someone stole something like this from you just so they could get a little cash.

But then you dissect it, and realize that person has some deep, unresolved scars that they may need help with. At the end of the day, I do not wish ill on this person, but hope that they have since found some healing and inner peace.

I personally don't think the baseball organization treated my situation justly. It was easy to see that they were just afraid to have a bad reputation due to how they would never directly answer any of my questions. There are security cameras at every corner of that place, so I know that they got footage of the person who took it; but still, they would always dodge my questions about the security footage when I asked.

Since my wheelchair was customized, it was pricier than a standard wheelchair. I sent the invoice from Missouri Vocational Rehab to the stadium coordinator, which said it was about $7,000, and the organization told me that it was too much money and that, if they needed to replace it, their budget would be way less than $7,000. That was mind-blowing to me. *It was stolen from* your *property after* your *employee said he would take care of it, and* you *won't replace what was taken from me? Where's your responsibility and owning your mistakes?* Plus they're an MLB franchise, and yet *my* wheelchair cost too much for their budget?!

Shame, shame, I know your middle name….

Due to complex implications like this in my life, when it came to dating, I was hardly expecting to meet someone new who could wholeheartedly and easily accept me for all of who I am. Someone who could even deal with what I had to deal with.

There were a lot of factors working against me that just didn't propel the whole dating-with-a-disability-and-a-kid thing forward, but I wouldn't know unless I tried…. So I took the plunge and signed up for some online dating apps. Honestly, I would so much rather just meet someone at a coffee shop or something, strike up a conversation, exchange numbers, and then begin the whole dating process that way; but in this day and age, online dating has topped the charts for ways to meet someone.

It's a weird process, if you dissect it: Put up some of your best pictures, write some things about yourself, and start "shopping." Let's be real, I bet the majority of people base their left and right swipes on looks alone. That seems to be the first thing most people look at right away; so, as a result, I decided not to include anything FA-related on my profile and didn't feature any pictures that showed a walker or wheelchair. It's more of a personal choice to disclose that information when the time feels right, anyways. I would never plan to meet someone in person without telling them, but I didn't want FA to be an immediate dealbreaker, or for someone to be quick to judge without giving me a chance and then pass me right up. I would hold off until I was comfortable to share. There are too many opinions we form—especially in the online arena—based on pictures alone. So I wanted to have the experience of connecting with someone and having a good conversation, organically—in the space before their assumptions about disabilities could set in.

Another reason why meeting someone out and about is so much better: You can see and feel their whole self, and pick up on their demeanor—even with just a quick conversation—when it's face-to-face.

Round 1 of signing up for the apps: I found the process to be pretty cool, actually. The platforms facilitate for a much larger dating pool and match you up with people that I, for one, probably wouldn't have the chance to cross paths with otherwise. For me, it was never about sleeping around or whatever negative stigmas there are around online dating; rather, it was in the hopes of finding a natural connection that could grow from that point forward.

Easier said than done, of course.

When I would share about my having FA with an online prospect, I was met with a slew of different outlooks and responses. I felt the time was right to share about my FA when we had expressed a mutual interest in meeting in person. I wouldn't dwell on it or speak negatively about it; I tried to brighten it up and be cheerful when sharing so that it all seemed less scary. I may have said: "I have something called Friedreich's Ataxia…" followed by some brief explanations; ending it with: "I would rather you not look it up because I know you're going to see the worst-case scenarios pop up first, and that's not typically me. I am an open book. If you have any questions, I'm happy to answer them and talk them through with you."

Either I would get a response like, "Wow, you're amazing," or "You have a great outlook and attitude;" or else I would get a, "Whoa, I wasn't expecting that. That's a lot of information, and I need time to digest." I would instantly know, at the latter response, that this was their way of speeding away and to not expect any more messages from them—I have been correct *every single time*.

Those who weren't bothered by it were very sweet and genuine, even if, in the end, we just didn't vibe, things just never flourished, or I could see they had different views of what FA would actually be like firsthand and freaked themselves out after date #1, so I never saw them again—unless these guys were just never that serious about a long term relationship from the get-go, if you catch my drift.

Most of our meetups were dates to get dinner together, a drink or both; even if things seemed to be going well, there was always that little voice in my head that reminded me not to get too gung-ho about it, because the chances of a second or even a third date were slim to none—see, I was starting to get familiar with the excuses that would usually follow a first date: "I'm so busy and have so much going on, maybe we can do something next week?!" Followed with no more calls or texts. "I'm not ready for a relationship." *Really? Because your profile read, "Looking for a serious relationship."* Or my favorite, "My dog chewed my phone, sorry I haven't been responding!" Followed with no calls or texts.

Seriously, guys?!

Like, is it just *me*—FA aside—that really is pushing you away? Or is it something to do with my disease? Sometimes it's one or the other or both and the shitty thing is, I'm not always sure and am left trying to figure out what the hell just happened! And that's the thing: I know it's not always the FA to blame. Like anyone who dates, feelings change and not all your dates or girlfriends or boyfriends will continuously be interested, or vice versa.

But the excuses are just so annoying. Just have the guts to say, "I'm just not that into you," or "I'm sorry but it's too much for me to consider dating someone in a wheelchair," and leave it at that. It'll sting, but it's like ripping off the band-aid, versus pulling it slowly to where I feel every tug. Those forceful and painful, dull conversations, asking or saying the worst thing or making something up of why they "suddenly" can't meet. I hate it!

Some actual messages I've received, to this effect:

- Can you, like, get dressed by yourself?
- Can you cook? Because I want a wifey to take care of me and not the other way around.
- Can you drive?
- Can you have sex?
- I want someone active—like, with their legs.
- We just aren't compatible.
- That's not what I am looking for.
- I am so sorry. You poor girl.
- I can't give you what you want or would need. *[What exactly is it that I need? Because you sure as hell never asked me!]*
- You won't be able to keep up with my lifestyle.
- I am sorry, I just can't handle this.

And my favorite of all time:

- We literally have this great connection already, but now that you told me this, I just don't know. I don't want to force feelings.

What does that even mean? Still can't crack that one.

I am not going to chase someone down to spell out my achievements and qualities if I am already being defined and labeled by my FA. I don't have much tolerance for those who judge a book by its cover.

Just in case, though, I made *sure* to create a beautiful cover for this book!

I will touch on one of the abovementioned taboo topics for a moment, though, since I know it to be something everyone wonders about. Sex: it's something you are probably curious about, but reserve on asking any disabled individual about because you're afraid it'll be offensive. Don't worry, I've got you… and yes, it is a *thing*, for sure. It can be a big thing, depending upon the person's specific questions, but I feel it should never be frowned upon to discuss it. We're all human and most have a sexual drive and desire—disability or not.

So. There are multiple ways to have kids these days, but I had mine the ole fashioned way. I'm hoping you can put two and two together that even though FA wasn't very apparent at the time my son was conceived, I still was diagnosed with FA and acted upon my inherent sex drive. And even as my diagnosis has progressed, sex is still a thing I love and explore. Maybe it's less so for me in particular, as I am not one to sleep with someone I'm not in a developed relationship with and am the kind of girl to "catch feelings," so it's definitely something meaningful to me. However, I want you to know that just because you tackle a disability, this doesn't mean sex is over. You can still have it and enjoy it! If positions have to be tweaked, then you tweak them.

Please, just never be embarrassed or ashamed for how your sex life needs to be. You only have one life, so enjoy yourself. Find and discover pleasure—it's only natural, and healthy. But remember this fine piece of advice: be responsible and be safe!

When you're online dating, there isn't even any physical contact yet, and still I experienced all these hardships and setbacks to what I thought would be an easy, or at least more enjoyable process. I thought it would be an easier way to get to know somebody. But eventually, the comments and complications drove me to a moment where I deleted my profile as fast as I could move my fingers to do so. I took some breathing room for a bit after that, but then eventually decided to give Round 2 a chance.

The same cycle, yet *again*! The struggle was trying to find guys who would take an interest in something other than my looks, followed by the ability to look past FA in order to get to know the *real me*. It was never easy. After Round 2 felt like it wasn't really going to work either, I took another break to regather my spirit. This was now starting to feel like a job, and I was exhausted, to be honest! I didn't think that trying to find a connection would bring so many excuses and so much *ghosting*.

Dating should be more fun and natural, not tons of work. Isn't the hard work supposed to be set aside for the marriage?!

It just turned out to be *such* an involved process. And there are a lot of steps to preparing someone to meet somebody like myself—starting from giving out all the necessary information, to worrying about how they will react, choosing a place to meet, and making sure it is handicap friendly. Typically it is, because a lot of things are accessible now, but there have been unforeseen instances before, and I would be a little apprehensive to want to ask assistance of somebody I'm meeting for the first time— especially romantically.

So there are physical stressors involved, too. It isn't just, *Are they going to like me?* or, *Am I going to like them?* When I used a walker, I would worry: *What if I fall? That would be embarrassing! Or what if I start choking? What if I spill my drink with my uncoordinated hand? What if I am having difficulty cutting my food? Do I ask for their help?* There are so many things that would circulate in my mind just around the symptoms of FA, that to add the typical first date jitters on top of that—Well, I'm only one person. I can only take so much.

Not to mention the struggles I face in just preparing to go out on a date in the first place. One time, I dropped my razor and couldn't bend down or find any sort of way to retrieve it, so I only had one shaven leg that night. I have since found a love for laser hair removal, even though it is in no way a cheap or painless process.

And I used to just let the leg hair go for a few days whenever I didn't feel like shaving, until one day, when Eli rubbed up on my prickly legs while we were telling stories lying down and said, "Ewww, that hurts, Mommy! It's like knives." I laughed while working to make peace with my prickly legs.

When I signed up for online dating yet again (*Third time's a charm, right?*) after a few months, I finally met someone who was wonderful. I hadn't felt this giddy about someone in a while, so it was nice to feel those butterflies again and to know that there were still gentlemen out there.

Matt and I both swiped right; once matched, we could message each other. He made it very easy for me to open up into having deep conversations pretty quickly. When we talked about meeting, I obviously told him about FA and he didn't bat an eye or shy away at all. It was so unbelievably awesome to not feel ashamed or unworthy of dating for once. We did a lot of what couples do and it was an eye opener that people with different abilities can, in fact, have wonderful relationships. Even though Matt's and my relationship didn't last more than three months, it was nice to feel like a part of the "normal" dating world—heartbreak of it ultimately not working and all.

A little less than a year later, I met Tim through some mutual friends, and we hit it off right away. I was a little nervous to open myself up to vulnerability again, but how do I know if a relationship will blossom if I don't try? We took ourselves out of the friend zone and made some enjoyable memories with trips to Florida and Hawaii. Looking back, Tim seemed to not let FA stand in the way, even though my physical needs were different than most people's. He was very conscious of my capabilities and knew when to step in. I really liked that. It meant a lot to me that he didn't complain and didn't mind lending a helping hand. Even though our relationship only lasted for four months, it served as a great reminder that not everyone you date will be "your person" or your "compatibility," even though they may be completely great. We dated and learned we weren't a great match, and that's just how the cookie crumbles sometimes.

Though disabilities can limit those interested in dating you, there exists also the possibility that you and your prospect just aren't going to jive with one another's personality, interests or hobbies, regardless.

It can be very discouraging to hear the same excuses and deal with someone who is less than what I deserve, but I can't change everyone's views on FA, wheelchairs, or differences in abilities. Though I surely will spread whatever awareness I can!

I've signed up for online dating a fifth, sixth and maybe seventh—I've lost count—time over the years, and found some really good guys interspersed amongst the typical judgmental ones. I think it's just going to be one of those things that I sign up for whenever I can handle it, and reside to love my single life when I don't want to be a part of it.

I'm still very much open to companionship and love, but I have also had to find peace in the possibility of not finding a long-term love. Maybe it's just not in the cards for me. Only God knows if the stars will align, but for now I'm doing me!

CHAPTER ELEVEN

Adaptations and Modifications

I am blessed to be able to keep trucking and that the world isn't as cruel as it once was. Don't get me wrong, it still is a bit inhumane, but organizations that have made it possible for someone like me to fit better into society have been a weight lifted off of the disabled community. Depending on the severity of your illness, injury, or impairment, it has been made possible for us to do more than just wither away inside the house.

I was very fortunate to benefit from Missouri Vocational Rehab in modifying my home, car, and receiving a wheelchair suited just for me! I am in awe of how organizations like this one really do make the biggest impact for the disabled community to strive to be as independent as possible.

I am not sure of the ins and outs of how each state runs their Vocational Rehab, but my home state of Missouri requires the individual to (1) have a physical, mental, emotional, or learning disability that is a real barrier to getting a job, (2) need Vocational Rehabilitation services to prepare you to get, keep, or regain employment, and (3) be able to benefit from the services that will assist you to get and keep a job or to benefit from independent living.

The timing couldn't have been more perfect for when I became connected with this offering. I had just started working for a wine company, doing sales in people's homes, as I was also getting ready to move into my parents' home, which is far from handicap friendly.

I needed my home to be equipped so that I could independently leave the house, get to work, and just live in general. It wasn't a quick process to getting approved, as there was a ton of paperwork, interviews, evaluations, measurements, etc. to compile and complete. After many months, I was given an ADA shower, a stair lift to go up and down the stairs, an outside deck lift to allow a smooth enter and exit process, hand controls for my car, a custom made wheelchair totally fitted for my body, and a topper on top of my car to carry my wheelchair while driving. It is amazing that I was eligible for this independence, but also sad to me that I need thousands of dollars of equipment just to function at home and when travelling. I knew that it was getting to be the time to transition my car to hand controls, though, so that I could safely drive for work and other personal purposes. Again, timing was on my side!

I feel I could write a whole book just on the adaptations and modifications I've had to make in my life in living with FA, but I'll try to narrow it down to just this chapter....

It wasn't like I woke up from a really bad accident one day and had to rely on a wheelchair from that day onward, so it's tough to see the whole picture of the changed capabilities of my day-to-day—mine have been progressing for over a decade.

Sometimes I do think, *What would it be like if FA were a disease that just hit you all at once, instead of little trickles for the rest of your life? Would it be easier to accept all at once? Would it be better to be paralyzed from the waist down, instead of having a genetic disease that affects the whole body? If I was, I wouldn't have to worry about passing my faulty gene onto my offspring. I'd have no problems speaking, or swallowing and choking. My torso and arms and neck wouldn't be lacking in coordination. I could have an unaffected upper body!*

I feel absolutely horrible for thinking these thoughts; and no one should compare, but come on! We're all human; I'm sure most of us have compared ourselves a time or two.

I know, realistically, nothing can change the fact that I've been given FA, but I can control the kind of person I am with FA. I choose not to feel ashamed for the help I can get. Or at least I try to—it's a work-in-progress. It has taken time, but I've come a long way from being stubborn against any assistance, to using a walker, to a wheelchair and all that came with that. And Missouri Vocational Rehab was the organization that really pulled through for me. I will always be grateful for them. The adaptations they've offered me have undoubtedly improved the quality of my day-to-day life.

As I was moving into my parents' place, the adaptations to the home took time, so in order to maneuver around the house, I had to go down the stairs on my butt, I had to have my mom help me in and out of her bathtub, I had to have someone bring my wheelchair up and down the stairs upon arrival or departure, and I had to share the bed with my mom (my dad sleeps in a different room because he snores louder than any human I know) as my room was still being prepped. I had to rely on rides for a few months, too, as it took me some time to grow the courage to drive my hand controls while I practiced in parking lots.

I had to adapt a lot more than just using a walker or wheelchair, though; it felt like every aspect of life was in a state of adaptation. I had to adjust to wearing clothes and shoes that required an easy slip on or pull over because buttons and zippers and clasps were becoming a real struggle. I had to adapt my hair style to it's naturally curly state because using a flat iron would require time, energy and much frustration. I found the importance of keeping snack-type foods in close proximity because I just couldn't reach the food on the top shelf in the refrigerator or the pot and pan too far back in the cabinet—I'd often just have to opt for chips and an apple as my dinner. I also adapted my room to where I had shelves at the wheelchair's level, so I could store my deodorant and lotions within easy grasp. And I grew the patience to take longer routes when driving because I realized quickly how I don't like to drive highways with hand controls, just side roads.

I have been blessed to where Missouri Vocational Rehab purchased and installed all of the adaptive devices in my home and car, and since I'm pretty sure most of you who are not so familiar with disabilities have no idea how costly it truly is to live disabled, I've decided to include a cost breakdown of all of my assistive mechanics:

- My customized wheelchair, designed to fit exactly to my body and to be used with the chair topper in my car: $7,072.23 (Some of these numbers are more precise, based upon my having easy access to the receipts.)

- My chair topper, that fits with my wheelchair and car: $4,256

- Hand controls for driving: $1,031

- A backup camera they built into my review mirror since my car doesn't have the screens built into it: $1,050

- Labor to do all this on my car: $1,430

- An outside wheelchair lift to go up and down from deck to ground that cost around $7000

- A stair lift inside my house to go up and down the stairs: these *start* at $10,000

- An ADA bathroom, including a roll-in shower with grab bars as well as grab bars around the toilet, and let's not forget the sub tile and the days of installation: over $5000

Add all that up and that's the amount I needed to be independent—somebody do the math—and move around my house without falling, drive my kid to school, and take a shower without assistance.

Look at these astronomical prices—all just to maneuver safely in my home and get from point A to point B. How is this ok? It makes sense how disabled folks seem to live simple and small, because we can't afford spacious homes, nice cars, expensive clothes and shoes, or the extracurricular things that would make our smiles bright, stomachs flat, faces glowing, vacations beautiful and relaxing, and spaces spruced up with the newness of buying power. Literally every penny counts. I save all my coins because I know building up to $10 will help me to put gas in my car.

I am fortunate to have had an organization cover the expenses of all my assistive devices, but I am on my own financially for any maintenance and replacements they require over time—which happens more than I would like.

Things break or need tune-ups, and even just one day without the lift can mean canceled plans because I'm stuck at home. Or if the power goes out from a storm, my stair lift and outside lift stop because they work off of electrical power. I better be downstairs if that happens, because if I'm not, I'll need to maneuver downstairs on my butt to use the bathroom.

It's those little things that turn into a big deal when the power is down, the weather is bad, or whatever small inconveniences come along to stop me in my tracks.

Friends and family really lighten the mood for me when I feel frustrated by it all. I find keeping them close helps to ward off any "woe is me" syndrome. I've even had two fundraisers put together by friends and family that granted me the financial assistance to be able to participate in research trials in another state, get necessary maintenance on my devices, and the option to be a part of FA events near and far.

The first fundraiser was held at a local restaurant with many silent auction baskets and raffles, and my friends created a GoFundMe account for those who couldn't attend but wanted to donate. I had never been in so much awe, just seeing all the support and all those who came to graciously give to me! Some were folks I hadn't seen in nearly ten years, and some were even unknown faces to me, but still supported me in some way. The second fundraiser was held two years later, when some family members and extended family organized a golf tournament fundraiser for me—and I had the glorious opportunity to be in awe again! Many familiar and unfamiliar faces, but all there to support and raise funds for little ole me!

I am humbled to have modifications and adaptations to make it easier for me to navigate my parents' home, but it surely would be nice if I had my own house to call home. I would have a home with no stairs. It'd be a totally handicapped-friendly home and I would be able to have every corner of my home the way I most prefer. If I had a home the way I see fit, I also wouldn't need two wheelchairs: one upstairs and one downstairs. I wouldn't need a stairlift or lift on the deck because I wouldn't have stairs. I would be able to set up the entire house to fit me optimally, instead of retrofitting my little apartment downstairs to make do.

My mom decorates in a really cute style, and I would say my taste is similar to hers, but it surely would be nice to take what I've learned from her and put it all into designing my own home. I remind myself to keep patience and that it will happen when the time is right.

CHAPTER TWELVE

FA Firsthand

Before I get into it, I want to make one thing crystal clear: I am *most* absolutely, without-a-*doubt* capable of mothering my child, despite every challenge and obstacle I may experience with FA.

Friedreich's Ataxia (FA), as you've gathered by this point, affects every part of my body and makes itself obvious by screwing up my movements in every way it can. The incoordination makes me look sloppy, intoxicated, weak, clumsy, awkward, and many more disgruntled adjectives, but you get the gist, so I'll leave it at that. Interpreting my own experience of my condition is sometimes hard—it can be difficult to get the words to really make sense of it, not to mention clearly differentiate what is me and what is my disease.

FA has affected my body to the point where pretty much every one of my movements or motions are *no longer* graceful. For example, not only am I making sure my arm, hand and fingers are grasping the remote control off the table enough to get the job done, but I am doing my best to keep my upper body from swaying all the while.

There've been times where Eli has said that I look like Master Splinter from the 1990's *Teenage Mutant Ninja Turtles* movie. It's the movement that looks sort of animatronic (i.e., robotic). Kind of stop-motion-animation like.

He's a kid, so I take this kind of comment lightly and of course don't take offense to it. However, Eli is a very transparent kid, so if he thinks I move like Master Splinter, I probably do, and other people may even see the same thing.

There are times where I could care less about being embarrassed by people staring and wondering about me; while other times, it really hits home. I've come to the realization that I mostly have a hard time if someone seems to feel I can't be trusted with their kids, pets, home, or anything else of inherent value—because I know wholeheartedly, I'm a trustworthy person, regardless of the limitations brought on by my FA. I know people are entitled to their own feelings towards someone, but when I am not chosen to be the protector of their valuables—AKA am viewed as untrustworthy because of my disability—I feel a bit hurt.

Why? I don't know. Perhaps it's just something I need to work on. Maybe their view of it isn't about me at all. Or maybe they don't want to feel like they're burdening me. Perhaps, since they aren't me, and they haven't had the experiences I've had in my own body, I just can't expect them to fully understand the scope of my capabilities, and that's ok. But hey, maybe it isn't okay that disabled people are judged unfairly in this capacity, too—myself included.

Still, every movement I make takes terrific concentration and I'm flipping tired just one hour after waking up because I needed to use full concentration and energy to submit to my morning routine. I have to transfer myself out of bed into the wheelchair, into and out of the restroom, then wheel myself to the stairs, transfer out of the wheelchair and into the stair lift, and then, once upstairs, transfer into a different wheelchair, have whatever caffeine is available so that I can function for the next hour and *then* start my day looking like a hot mess either to drive Eli to school, or just to accomplish the other millions of responsibilities that I have. Honestly, no day looks the same—other than maybe my crazy hair—except for when I have Eli and we have to get him to school.

We like a good routine for that, because I'll tell you what: School mornings are *chaos* without routine. The alarm is set for 6:00 am (Eli's ideal choice of time) and we're headed out the door by 6:55 am. *Heading out the door* isn't your typical "jumping in the car" for us, though. I have to leave through the back door on the deck, wheel myself to the chair lift, get on, push the button to go down, wheel off, type in a code (which hardly works) to open a gate, wheel myself to the car, transfer to the driver's seat, take the seat cushion off the wheelchair, fold it in half, bring the hook down on the chair topper, hook the chair, bring it up, start my car, engage the hand controls and... we're off, *finally*! However, since I don't like to drive the highways with my hand controls, I opt to take the longer, more scenic route. Eli's school is between a twenty-three to thirty-two minute drive, depending on traffic, so after I drop him off, I head to my "office," which is a subdivision street down the road where I can park myself and check my emails, my schedule, and map out my to-do list for that day.

Once I get home, I sometimes need to get myself ready to go out in public, which should probably require a shower, putting on clothes that aren't my PJs, and maybe a brush to my hair and swipe of makeup to my face; which, let's be real, probably won't happen... it's just wishful thinking. All of the things I need to do to even look like a decent human being tire me out like no other. A shower isn't just a quick scrub and wash; it's a full-blown job. The only way for me to independently shower—something that means so much to me, that I never could've thought I'd one day be *so* thankful for—is to use a shower chair to sit on while I wash. I am so grateful for this piece of equipment that allows me to shower all by myself, rather than requiring the help of someone else to do so.

I am still able to stand and transfer out of a wheelchair in the bathroom with the use of my grab bars, so thankfully I do not need to use my wheelchair in the shower or have to worry about drying it off. Once in the shower, it is no longer a second nature part of life, though; I need to be on full alert to not move in any sort of speedy manner that could result in my falling out of the chair, and I need to make sure to fully grasp the bottles of shampoo and conditioner, so they don't slip out of my hands.

If, by chance, that does happen, then there's a 50/50 shot I'll be able to pick them back up and retrieve them. I have to find a very safe way to bend down and reach them, or else I can end up toppling out of the whole situation. And you know well by now the terror of my razor blade troubles. But even when brushing my teeth, I've dropped the toothpaste bottle under my sink, unable to reach it, and have had to just grab Eli's bubblegum toothpaste to do the job. It's the things we usually take for granted that are the tasks I need to *work* for.

My days are filled with constant reminders that I will have to do *extra* to complete a task. FA has taken my abilities and shrunken them down. I feel like I'm constantly weighed down by heavy weights strewn all across my body, and I have to use lots of strength and tons of concentration to coordinate my arm just to grab my jacket and awkwardly put it on. I have to use arm strength to wheel myself to the kitchen table even when I'm too tired at the thought of picking up a fork—eating and most likely dropping the fork repeatedly is an exhausting cycle! Even though some days it's very enticing to just stay in bed and sleep, I not only have to be up and moving for my son, but I *want* to be. I want to be the mom who pushes through the obstacles, in the hopes that my son grows up to have the same kick-ass mentality. *Who* said life would be easy? That's a question I constantly remind myself of because putting in the work means I'm not letting FA win—and FA will *never. fucking. win.*

The first word that comes to mind when I think of having FA is "work." It takes work just to stay alive, which at times feels unfair. As much as I hate using the "unfair" word, it is truthfully how I feel some days. The world isn't as handicapped friendly, as accessible, as you may think. Yeah, *sure*, to an outsider looking in, there's ramps, elevators, assisted devices, handicap bathroom stalls, home modifications, disability checks… but is it enough? Enough to make navigating the world easier? Akin to being able-bodied? *Hell* no.

Do you realize how much money disabled individuals need to spend out of pocket to do the things the average Joe can do for $0?! I have to fork up big bucks just to be part of the society. And I just—I don't think that's fair. There are organizations and scholarships and fundraisers to help, but not everyone benefits. I feel there should be some other support. Wouldn't it be nice if the government accommodated *every* disability?! I mean, why do we need to spend countless days, weeks, and months asking, fighting, appealing, and filling out pages of documents—just to simply move around the home as an able-bodied person would?

The disease, now, I can't do much about that, except for show up to fight it as best I can each and every day, take part in research trials, and attend fundraisers. But finances seem to be such a simple problem to solve, if only funds were dispersed in a more effective and ergonomic way. They're something I may be able to do something about. Or, if not me, then somebody. I just don't understand why not only the cards, but the bills are stacked against the disabled.

Sometimes it honestly feels like I'm being punished by this disability. Like, did I have a past life where I royally pissed people off, so I've had to come back and experience *this* as my punishment? It may sound crazy, but I've wondered through every rabbit hole.

Most of the time, I find positivity in my misfortune, because in the realness of life, I know that so many other people are going through *something*. Something that brings them to the brink of their own being. The world isn't designed to where everyone is the same, which is precisely where I come in… I feel I am designed to show and explain my difference; that being FA.

Yes, FAers are always going to have to work their asses off, but it is possible to be a parent. It's possible to have a relationship, a family, a career… go to school, be independent—but it does and will come with hard challenges. Uphill battles you fight every day to ascend.

FA feels like a disease meant to kill its victims—but don't let it! Don't you *dare* let it.

There seems to be a double-edged sword to every mishap. Let's taking eating, for example: First it destroys my balance and coordination, so I have to use a wheelchair. It messes up my dexterity and sensation, causing me to drop my fork on the ground, due to the sensation loss of the fingers that were holding it. Then I need to maneuver in a strange manner to bend over and pick up the fork, all while feeling unsteady like I may topple out of my chair, my coordination so poor that I have a hard time even aiming my fingers in the correct direction. Once I finally do grab it, I lift my upper body upwards, whack my head on the table on the way, spill my glass of water and then run into the problem of not being able to reach the paper towels on the counter. I assess the area to see if I can safely stand up without totally eating dirt, and luckily, I'm able to hang on to the sink for support to stand. Only, I need to release one hand to reach for the paper towels, so I need full concentration to not lose balance and wipe out. Once I get them, I need to wipe up the mess, again trying not to fall out of my chair.... Should all of this go well, we consider it a success!

But now, here I have spent twenty-five minutes picking up a fork and cleaning a mess, and never even got to enjoy my meal. Now I have an obligation at this time, have to get ready or leave the house, and can't eat. I'm hungry and thirsty, but definitely can't do either while driving with my hand controls. All I have time for is to grab a bottle of water and take sips at red lights when I put the car in park to free up one hand for all of ten seconds. I better not drink too much, though, because then I'll have to pee, and I can't tell you how many times I've run—again, an operative word—into a gas station's accessible bathroom only to find crates of food covering half the path, an "out of order" sign on the door, or have spent time I don't have to waste waiting for the one accessible bathroom to become vacant. And how much do you want to bet that an able-bodied person is using it because it's so *spacious*?

FA wants to win and no matter how much I fight back, it's still in the lead. It isn't treatable, so it is always just a matter of time before it progresses further, and further, and further.... But treating this son of a bitch is exactly what needs to happen, because it is damn scary what this beast is capable of. Destroying hearts, which leads to cardiomyopathy. Diabetes. Injuries from falls. And just the mind-numbing persecution of needing to focus so diligently on every action and on every single movement.

If you let it completely take over, it will strip you from society completely. No friends. No socialization. Just existing—not living. But that's the scariest for me. I need to keep friends and family close, to keep some positivity alive. Some hope for the future. Hope for myself.

Having FA, basically, feels like not having much control over my body. And losing more control every day, no matter what I do. For example, when I go to the gym, Lisa, my trainer, has me get up and walk around—holding her hands of course. I can feel *everything*, every stretch, shift, resistance and ache, and I just have a very difficult time moving how I'd like to. Having to initiate the motion of walking is just so hard. Picking my foot up to move it forward seems simple, but my nerve endings don't talk and signal like they should, so I have to really give my concentration to get my feet and legs to move. Though when I do get them to move, it is slow and sloppy looking. I need to concentrate on moving my lower extremities while my torso and hips are swaying, which only makes it harder to keep my walking posture intact. And between each step, I need to switch my mind back over, to concentrate again on keeping my upper body from going all over the place.

All the while, I mantra to myself: "Keep your core tight, look up, keep a straight posture and don't forget to breathe!" Then I have to switch gears again and tell my other leg to lift up and take a step forward. And so on and so forth.

Whew! Just explaining it is exhausting! I am just about wiped after ten steps.

Getting into bed is a job too. Lifting myself up and grabbing the fitted sheet to keep from falling over (not the safest maneuver) and then lifting one leg into bed, followed by the other, where I more often than not topple over in the bed—and to then move my body into the proper place is like moving five hundred pounds. Getting my limbs to work together seems impossible, so one by one, I move an arm for stability, then a leg for support, then the other arm, and then the last leg. Turning over to my back and moving side to side isn't just a simple body roll—no—I've got to sit up and use my arms to push me over to one side.

Good thing I'm already in bed—I'm exhausted! And are you, dear reader? Exhausted by the sound of my daily life? Exhausted by the tests I face, by the feeling of lead in your bones and an uncooperative body system? I kinda hope so. I hope you can empathize with the burden of this condition. I hope you feel my pain. Because as much as I like to try to stay positive and clear about my purpose, I am in pain. I am struggling to survive; to fight this doom of a disease as it tries to destroy me.

And no, I wouldn't wish this on even my most hated enemy. I hope you never have to actually experience the breaking, the dismantling of your physical body. And if you do, or if you have FA, even, my heart swells in love for your struggle… for your pain. I *feel* you. I am you.

CHAPTER THIRTEEN

Counseling

I love counseling! Seriously, it is so great to get everything off your chest, even if it doesn't make a lick of sense to you. Counseling may get that taboo reputation we've all heard, but I hope more people take the opportunity to invite it in. To let it help. Counseling has given me so much insight in dealing with my overwhelming life hardships. Even just having somebody neutral to talk to, and to get feedback from on whatever I'm moving through… it's priceless!

Counseling was, actually, the career path I had originally wanted to pursue, so I knew the benefits and, after Matt and I had broken up, figured I should practice what I preach. So I gave it a whirl, but after a few sessions, wasn't getting close to any sort of bond with the therapist. She was old school and didn't come at all close to jiving with what I was sharing. The room just felt cold. And with that, please turn to lesson one: Not all counselors or therapists will be a great fit for you! I believe a good, healthy connection needs to be established between you and your therapist if you're going to reveal all the ins and outs of your life.

I ended my sessions with the cold lady, and instead, turned to using a lot of relationship tools I had learned throughout the years, alongside advice offered from loved ones. Eventually, and quite quickly actually, I got back on a good path and felt confident in my life with Eli, FA, co-parenting, friendships, dating… you name it, everything seemed to be smoothly sailing along.

It was about eighteen months after that first therapist meeting when I began counseling again. I was having a hard time with many aspects of life: between my progressing symptoms, dating life, unresolved emotions, new physical challenges, and just figuring it all out, I felt overwhelmed. This time around, though, counseling just kind of fell into my lap, for a lack of better words.

The process started when I signed Eli up for counseling. I wanted him to go, as many dynamics in his life were twisting and changing rapidly at the time. My hope was for Eli to feel he had a place to be free to just talk, in case there was something he didn't really want to dive into with Joey or myself. He, maybe, went for a handful of sessions when I learned he did not really need it. I am very fortunate to have a pretty open and honest relationship with Eli, and he hasn't been shy to talk with me about pretty much anything—at least for now. We have definitely strengthened our relationship and bond by talking, active listening, and by my giving him advice and encouragement when we do.

Anyway, when I would bring him to the office and wait in the waiting room, I would read a lot of the signs and pamphlets about adult counseling for separated / divorced parents and the benefits of it. Most Co-Parents struggle, no matter the situation, but mine in particular just felt so difficult to grasp, and my thought process around it all felt so confused. Like I couldn't quite make peace with it. So it was time for a different approach: to surrender to an outsider helping. I felt like I was always doing my best, but I still had doubts. Doubts that I wasn't being the mother Eli deserved. Doubts that others didn't think I was someone to take seriously. Doubts about navigating legalization in the child custody realm. Doubts about how a positive future would look. Doubts around how FA can play into motherhood, friends, family, a partner and just life in general.

I wasn't in the super-depressed, sleeping-all-day, not-socializing phase, but I was hoping to snap out of my 'doubtful' limbo *before* I full-blown got there. You don't need to hit rock bottom to seek help! That's why I think counseling / therapy gets a reputation for people only going when they have tons of problems or psychiatric conditions or addictions… but you can go just to straighten things out in your life before they go completely sideways. I do feel the self-improvement game becoming more and more mainstream, though, which just feels right! Take care of yourself! Yes! *Thank you.*

I sent an email to the counseling service. Now, Eli only went that handful of times, but once I got started, I went weekly for two years. When I sent the email, I explained my need for counseling and was matched to a therapist who was a great fit. And he *was* the perfect fit. I have so much gratitude for this therapist—he's helped me tremendously!

I seriously was excited for this journey after connecting with my new therapist; I knew it couldn't make matters worse, and I was ready to put in the right effort—the effort of showing up and being open and honest. You can't accept help if you're shut down and unwilling!

Counseling is definitely not a quick fix, though. It takes time to build that trust with your therapist; I wanted to be there, so it wasn't like pulling teeth to get me to participate. But it wasn't like I just *ripped the band-aid off*, either. Having the patience to work on yourself is key; sure, it's a bit weird and awkward at first, but once those walls get broken down, it gets a whole lot smoother.

The doubts I was experiencing coupled well with patterns of putting myself down; they pretty much all linked together. I was filled with questions on where I stood as a mother because I am a single one, and one with physical limitations, to boot. It's probably something I will have ups and downs with the whole journey through, but remembering to *do the best I can with the deck of cards I've been handed,* and *to set boundaries* have been great mottos of guidance for me. I have been able to acknowledge and feel pride in my capabilities and in doing what works best for Eli and me—rather than compare myself to other parents. I'm not that mom who enforces their kid to sleep in his bed. I'm not the mom who prepares—or, to have my mom prepare and cook—a home cooked meal by 5:30 every night, either. I'm not the mom who says, "Only thirty minutes of screen time per day," nor am I that mom that follows a strict schedule. But I sure as hell show endless love to my kid, enforce good and safe choices, and encourage him to definitely not sweat the small stuff. I have learned to set the bar to my level which has allowed for a better parenting relationship, and it shows I can follow through with my rules for Eli. I choose to provide security in regards to his expectations of me, so he knows what he is getting and can trust in that.

I used to put myself down for having to sit on the sidelines, instead of being able to run around and kick the ball with Eli. But I learned to find the joy in watching and cheering and trying new limits to see where I am capable of tweaking my involvement.

I've found a new appreciation for doing what I can, like playing board games, reading, playing action figures on the ground, watching movies and our all-time favorite: talking and sharing stories. I've instilled how important talking and listening are, and I always promise to listen and give sound advice, instead of scolding him or getting upset. I think it is very important to teach your kids and give explanations rather than just saying, "No!"

I used to have a hard time accepting my mom's help in making Eli's school lunches and dinner, but acknowledging her selfless act to do these things for us has allowed me to concentrate on the bigger stuff, like driving Eli to and from school, helping with his homework and spending quality time I might otherwise miss out on, were my mom not helping out.

Joey and I share parenthood over the same child, so if he didn't necessarily like what I was doing, it would put me in a mentality where I'm somehow in the wrong. I guess I was losing confidence in myself at the time as a result of these ways of thinking. Counseling helped me shift this perspective to where I no longer put either Joey or myself in the wrong. What I have learned is how Joey and I just hold different beliefs, and thus use different techniques—techniques that we each believe are what's best for us. Since we are not together or living under the same roof, it is perfectly okay for each of us to do what works for us, separately, in raising Eli. We do not need to have dinner the same way and at the same time. Eli can have a different routine with homework and playtime. He may have different bedtimes and nightly routines. Eli may have different, fewer, or more chores at one house versus the other. Different ways in different environments.

It's a fine line, to discern how Eli actually feels about living this way with the different households, to make sure he's fully comfortable at both, but I'd honestly say he is. He understands things are a little different from mom's to dad's, and he has adapted with neutrality.

Counseling helped me to realize that these differences were actually totally okay, because our son's needs are fully met. My therapist would always remind me that I cannot have control over what goes on at his dad's, and Joey can't at my house, either. I'm not there and he's not here. "You can only control what you can do and be." This has helped me… more than I can say! I lost a lot of the anxiety just in reframing this view of myself as a parent. In turn, this has given me confidence in my role as a mother, even with my limitations; and actually, because of FA, how much more I appreciate the bond and closeness I have with Eli.

Therapy shifted me into understanding my importance and thus doubting myself less. I learned to use boundaries and how to keep the peace, even when there were disagreements between Joey and myself as Co-Parents. Placing boundaries in life is gold! Don't mistake my boundaries as walls, though—a wall is firm and inflexible, while a boundary can be altered depending on the situation.

CHAPTER FOURTEEN

Adapting to a Pandemic with FA

ERIN K PIEPER

U nless you've been living under a rock, you should be familiar with the recent global pandemic of Covid-19 that has shaken the earth.

When many areas of the world went into lockdown, I became faced with a sense of relief, honestly. I'm neither a homebody nor one who enjoys seclusion for long periods of time, so that part was hard, but knowing I didn't have to worry about the complications of needing assistance to attend the usual flow of concerts, sporting events, parties, weddings, showers, and such was a nice break. See, for me to attend any kind of event that takes driving, walking, entrances and exits, public restrooms, etc., it can become a full-on checklist. I enjoy big events, but I usually have to be on the radar to make sure I either have someone who can help out if need be or just ensure that I did my homework so things [hopefully] are smooth sailing. So, there was that part of ease for me in navigating the pandemic.

I wish I didn't have to feel that way, though. I'd very much like to just freely walk and skip along to a baseball game or a night out on the town without worrying about getting a parking spot close to an entrance with no stairs. I'd love it if I didn't have to stress when the one and only accessible bathroom is out of order, or the careless able-bodied person is using it for its spacious luxury.

Food for thought: What if the world was majority handicapped and the minority was able-bodied? Or what if the world was designed to support and facilitate ease for handicapped people, and the able-bodied folk navigated *that* world? I feel this would be an apt and fertile world; one ripe with consideration for those less privileged.

"We're in this together," and "these challenging times" are two phrases that kind of make me cringe. I may sound like an a-hole, but what I want to say is coming from a good place. Ever since I was diagnosed with FA, life has been challenging. I don't want to overstep, and I don't want to put words in the mouths of those who have a disease, disability, or life-changing illness, but I bet some of you can relate to this. I've overcome many obstacles and challenges, but with FA they don't vanish once you overcome them. You don't get a gold medal for achieving them. There isn't any camaraderie of "we did good, team." No. It's just you, accepting and surrendering to your circumstances without giving up hope or stopping the fight. You put in so much work just to relieve some back pain and get a good night's rest. Then the challenges reset and you have to overcome them *again* the next day—and all the while, it may get harder and harder each and every time.

For me, it's challenging *all the time*—with or without Corona.

Having freedoms stripped away, much like what we all experienced and still are somewhat, isn't all that new to me. I've been stripped of things since well before Covid, and will continue to be stripped of them after. Tweaking things in order to be creative at the home, again, is nothing new to me. Letting go of your career even though you don't want to… yep, been there. Dealing with financial distress—bills, groceries, hobbies, kids… welcome to my life *way* before this virus. Pulling your hair out from dealing with the government, filling out applications, being a needle in the haystack, waiting, waiting, waiting for financial assistance… I have dealt with this for years, every few months, and will continue to deal with this—this is, unfortunately, my norm.

Being told, "No," or, "You're not the candidate we're looking for," or, "I'm sorry," are words I always hear, so nothing new here.

Having to redirect your kid(s) into doing activities with you and staying home… it's not always easy; trust me, I get it! Because of my limitations in being able to "run" around with Eli, I don't take what I *do* get to do with him for granted: drawing together, playing board games, storytelling, reading, watching movies together, being by his side when he plays sports in the backyard, teaching cooking skills, talking about real life shit… it's just the way it is.

I mean, if I (and many others) face and deal with this on the regular—like *all* of what's been brought on by this pandemic—then why *now* is it we're "all in this together"? It took a virus for people to say this? Why couldn't we be in these challenges *together* before? I bet this slogan will not hold after Corona, but why *don't* we stand together when the nation [after COVID-19] will still have many cancer sufferers, mental health issues and deaths? Many untreatable diseases and disabilities? Addictions? Diabetes? Heart disease? Suicide? The list goes on…. So, why don't we strive to keep the slogan strong, and remember how much stronger we are together, when we share our challenges and are there for each other.

As a not-so-sidenote, healthcare workers and first responders and all those working their tails off to save lives (COVID or otherwise) should *always* be appreciated and applauded—not just now. And I don't mean a donation of money here and there to organizations, which is always a nice gesture, but I mean the blood, sweat and tears of really being in this together. True, actual support. The support and prayers and love that is being poured during this pandemic should be continuously poured out, ever after!

So basically, the world, the people, situations, diseases, and deaths are extremely challenging life issues we all face, regardless of COVID, and I hope people realize to continue to be in it *all* together, *all* the time. We are all always going through something, and so can you imagine just how strong our world would be if we *always* supported one another like we are now. I can, and it's beautiful.

CHAPTER FIFTEEN

Research Trials

I started my very first clinical trial at USF, the University of South Florida, in 2013. I felt compelled to take part in research and clinical trials from the get-go, as I am so passionate about doing what I can to support finding a treatment or cure for Friedreich's Ataxia.

Basically, the way these trials work is that you add your name and info to a database on the FARA website so that whenever spots open up in a trial, they can connect with you to conduct a screen visit, where they collect blood work, inquire about the prognosis of your FA or it's progression, as well as your age, gender, whether you're pregnant.... All these factors come into play with whether you would be a good fit for their current trial or not. They may ask you to ride a stationary bike or walk down a hallway to test your capabilities and see whether your capabilities are in their ideal window for test subjects.

One test I always remember is called the Nine-Peg-Hole Test, where they put this little thing in front of you that has nine holes in it, and then they hand you nine pegs. They want to see how fast you can fill the holes with the pegs, one hand at a time, and then they ask you to take them out. Now, I know it may not *sound* like much, but this task is super annoying and super tedious because it tests your dexterity and coordination. It really is just not a pleasant test to take, but it seems to be one of the best tells for where you're at with the progression of your FA.

Once you start taking medication for whatever trail you become a part of, they will regularly have you do these same tests, to see whether the medicine is having any impact on your symptoms or progression.

After the screening, they'll typically come back a few days later with either a confirmation that you're the right fit for the trial, or they will deny your admittance. If you are accepted, they'll send packets of information for you to peruse as you decide whether you want to do it, take the meds, and the whole nine yards. You have about a thirty-day window before you begin the study you have accepted. I typically say yes to doing all the ones they call the Safety and Tolerability tests; meaning, the meds have already been tested in the lab, but it's the first time they've been tested on a human, so they want to see if it's safe and tolerable for human use.

The only ones I've been a part of have had super minimal side effects; I'm pretty particular about not choosing anything that could cause a lot of side effects or a lot of unknowns. The typical ones where maybe a slight headache, nausea, or constipation is all you risk, those are the ones I'll do; but anything much bigger than that—I remember there was one that said it could cause kidney or liver damage, or even death—yeah, no thanks.

The beginning of the trial is easy-peasy, but then when you take the meds that first day, there's a window of time before you have a follow-up screening, and the windows tend to get longer and longer as the trial progresses. So it may be the case where you go there for a day to start the trial, then go back 7 days later for the day, then come back another 10 days later, and so on for the duration of the trial. I'll probably make about four trips in a thirty-day trial. My mom generally accompanies me, and we'll travel down the night before to go get something to eat and squeeze in as much R&R as we can before I go in for the trial the following day. Then we'll go shopping, go see a museum, or do whatever we want to do before we leave the following afternoon.

I've taken part in about seven, maybe eight, rounds of these trials so far. And I always opt to do the ones at USF in Tampa. They're like family there to me by now, and they will casually ask me, nowadays, whether I want to take part in an upcoming trial. I'll just get a text or call, and we'll move into the screening process from there.

I like that all my trials take place in this one location; it's like a second home to me, we've been doing it for so many years now. There are other locations, one in Philadelphia, one in LA, but I just don't feel like having to get to know a whole new travel routine. We know all the ins and outs of that area, we just love Florida anyway, and it's such a quick, two-hour flight.

I will say that, over the years, it's gotten a bit taxing to travel there and back so much. I come home, mother my Eli, go back, and so on. And it never bothered me until now, I feel mostly because I'm progressing to the point where I'm tiring more easily, and also due, perhaps, to the up and down from the plane, getting to the hotel, and having to navigate all that with the wheelchair…. I'm starting to become more selective; more trusting of my intuition on whether or not I'm meant to do a particular trial.

It is cool to be a part of this stuff, as it could potentially benefit me to learn what could improve my experience. I want to do them not only for myself, but for the community of FAers; however, I am a mother, and have Eli to think about, so I feel that takes precedence in my life, every day in every way. I feel I was sort of saved by the bell with Covid forcing me to slow down and realize how taxing the trials can actually be for me.

During the trials, they want you to document everything—and I mean everything, from sneezing to an odd sensation to a weird bowel movement—so they can then compare notes between all the participants. Sometimes, there are dietary restrictions—once, I couldn't eat anything with PUFA (polyunsaturated fatty acids), which is shockingly in everything, and my diet was so light at that time as a result. I believe I lost ten pounds, without trying, in thirty days. I'm already a small girl, so I finished the trial looking like I was fifteen years old again!

Sometimes they give you a placebo, and honestly, sometimes I'm not sure whether I'm receiving it or not. I'm like, *Was that a symptom of the drug? Or was that just me?*

Most of the time, the coordinators at the university will set up your car rental, hotel, and flights. Other times, they'll have a travel agent set it up for you. Now, I like Southwest because I can preboard and can pick my own seat. So this way, I can navigate to where I'm comfortable without feeling the stress of holding others up behind me, or needing to sit uncomfortably for the flight because I got stuck in an awkward seat for me to have to sit in. My wheelchair for travel is super slim, so even though it cannot fit the whole length of the plane, I can generally maneuver it through the aisle of the first few rows easily enough. And I also like how Southwest has a straight flight from St. Louis to Tampa, and it's super speedy and easy to only have to work my way around one plane.

So I generally will research my ideal flights and send the info over to the coordinators at the university's travel agent office. Generally, this is not a problem. With hotels, I've run into a few issues and have learned to work them out. Especially if you book an ADA room.

An ADA room should be set up for accessibility, ADA-equipped with handlebars around the toilet, a lower sink, a roll-in shower with a bench built-in, and have ample space to navigate a wheelchair. Sometimes, the rooms are perfect, and the setup is super helpful and easy to traverse. Other times, not so much. The worst thing I've encountered is with the showers. The ADA showers or bathtubs are just very different depending on the hotel. Some must feel they're ADA compliant just by putting grab bars in the bathtub. With that, though, I still have to step into the bathtub. And then I need to sit, but there's obviously nowhere for me to sit, so the grab bars are not going to be that helpful for me.

I've also had it where they just give me a roll-in shower. However, I don't roll my wheelchair in there because it's the only one I've got with me while travelling, so I don't want to get it soaking wet. They typically have a shower bench in those rolling ones, though, so I am more able to shower in those, where I can pivot my way from my wheelchair over to the shower bench.

I've voiced numerous times, when I run into ADA issues, to whoever is booking my room, that they need to be aware of what sort of room accessibility a hotel provides—especially since these trials are for drugs to assist the *disabled*. And of course, there are the verbal apologies yet again; they thought everything was hunky-dory, but it wasn't. So I've just learned that, once I get the confirmation email from whoever's booking my room, I must call the hotel and triple check and say something like, "Here I am, here's my confirmation number…. So what's the room you have me in? What's it look like? How is it equipped?" If it's something that doesn't work for me, then I need to be vocal with them about what I need; and typically it isn't an issue, as they can just move me into what I do need. But I've learned my lesson: I've gotta do what I've gotta do. Sometimes you've just got to take matters totally into your own hands!

All but one trial I've done reimbursed all meals, gas, and any other travel costs. Which, honestly, is necessary in order for me, and most likely most of those who attend, to even be able to take part in the trials. That first trial, however, did not compensate or pay for anything. Luckily for me, however, my friends and family helped out with donations, and then a year or so later, the first fundraiser was thrown and helped me with the future visits.

And it is really rewarding to me to be a part of these trials. Even though it is taxing travel time for me, the other side of the coin is that, if there's going to be medication out there, and they need to figure out how it's gonna work, I am thrilled to be a part of that!

Back when I first started partaking in trials, I checked all the boxes and was pretty gung-ho on doing everything myself, being independent, and fighting my disease as best I could. I thought, *If I can do it all, then I need to do this.*

I feel like there was this little voice that said, "You know what? This is your time to shine; your time to do what you can for this challenge to become easier for anyone who follows you, and so you need to do it."

And it is rewarding. These doctors, researchers, nurses, scientists, whatever; they need participants so we can try to find something helpful.

And now, realistically, I do not think—and I'm trying not to be a Debbie Downer here; I'm just realistically speaking from where I'm at with my age and prognosis right now—I don't necessarily think there's going to be this absolutely amazing treatment for me, in my lifetime. But I do believe that there can be something for later generations, after me. People who maybe are being newly diagnosed right now, are not very far in their prognosis, a lot younger in life, or don't really have any other medical conditions that go along with that…. I really do feel that I can benefit them. And so I do my best to just be happy about that.

And I want to say, I'm pretty okay and happy with that truth. I mean, yeah, I get moments where I'm like, *How wonderful would it be if, in five years, you know, I just got up and I started walking and could talk better and move better, and be more available and do a lot more as a mom, and just as a person in general?* Like, I'm sorry, people can sit there and just accept what their disability is, but if someone were to come up to you and say, "I have a magic pill for you, the curing treatment!" You'd say, "Ummm, absolutely!" without hesitation. I don't know one person who would say, "No, I like being in a wheelchair. I like sleeping all day." *No*, absolutely not.

There are generally three stages to drug trials before they can go to apply for approval with the FDA. Now, sometimes I get a little skeptical that the trials will ever really go anywhere. I often wonder if the pharmaceutical companies *actually* want us to get better, or whether they aren't as moral as we wish they were, and instead stand to benefit more when drugs aren't trying to be a *cure*. However, I know that the world is changing—I see it—and still take part in these trials because I am hoping for the best, and mostly so for the younger generations who may come to face this terribly challenging diagnosis.

My heart is with them. My efforts are for them.

CHAPTER SIXTEEN

Inspiration

The meaning of "inspiration," according to the online dictionary, basically means something that makes someone want to do something or that gives someone an idea about what to do or create.

Now, I'm sure most of us can relate to going on Pinterest to get inspired in handcrafting or cooking or styling or pretty much anything, just to get our juices flowing on a project or idea. Perhaps it's watching videos and movies, reading a book, or hearing someone share their life experiences that has shifted your mind in wanting to do better or has inspired you to be some kind of superhuman, in whatever way. Possibly, you feel inspired by your spouse, kids, family members, or friends to do better, or be better. No matter how it's been embedded, I am sure many people have found inspiration in their life in one way or another.

I am often told, "You're such an inspiration, Erin," or, "I want to be a better person because of you," or, "You're so brave...."

But what is it that makes me an inspiration to someone?

Is it because I embody a way of being that someone wants to follow? Is it my strength? Or is it because I am an optimistic, pushing-my-limits, not-giving-up wheelchair user? Or that I am not only confident in myself, but in others reaching towards a greater good?

I get inspired from other folks who have been diagnosed all the time. Among the ranks, I find all sorts of inspiring, innovative ideas for making life easier or better. I don't know how to label it exactly, but I like whatever they're doing, and I want to incorporate whatever it is into my own life. Like that wheelchair user who found a way to clip a water bottle on the bar of their wheelchair—genius. Or that woman who's wearing shorts that look like they button up, but really it's an elastic band holding the shorts up?! Amazing.

I guess it depends on what "inspiration'" means to you. I've always liked to use the word "motivation" when describing "inspiration," but with some research I've come to see how motivation is more aimed towards external rewards, and inspiration, on the other hand, starts from within and is an intrinsic reward.

So inspiration really just means you soak up a good idea and then put in the work to make it come to fruition in your own life. Or someone else's idea gives you another, different and exciting idea.

All I'm really doing is just spreading those little light bulbs in people's minds, but I love to believe that that's what I'm doing when I aim to be my best self. I think it's pretty cool and truly humbling that someone would look to incorporate my doings in their life for better outcomes. That anyone could find me an inspiration.

I like to believe I've been given this unfortunate disease to shed some positivity and use my voice to encourage myself and others toward brighter days. FAers have to work quadruple as hard to do the things society deems "normal," and that is where the idea of being an inspiration to others makes me gloat. If I can tackle the millions of responsibilities in my world, then I want to show others they can tackle their own life responsibilities too, with the ideas that I share.

I've heard from other FAers and disability advocates alike that being called "an inspiration" isn't something they particularly appreciate. I do understand this side of it, too. There are some people who simply say it because they don't know what else to say. Like—are you *truly* inspired and moved? Are you going to go home from work and start incorporating my thoughts, actions, and energy into your life? Or are you just saying it because Susie Q said it to a disabled individual, and it sounded so nice when she did?

To be fair, though, this probably occurs only because the world has shown us that disabilities are a life full of sadness, and that we should pat the backs of handicapped individuals everywhere because they are "exceptional" and a "force to be reckoned with" for going on with their lives. In all honesty, I and other people who are faced with a handicap are just doing the best that we can with the hand we've been dealt. Just because I am using my body to the best of its capability, I do not feel I deserve an achievement award or a standing ovation; I simply like knowing that someone tried my hack of working out in a wheelchair to incorporate it in their life for themselves! I don't think I need a gold medal for figuring that one out—however, I will take it, if you're offering!

In all seriousness, if they feel and think I'm an inspiration, then I'll let them feel and think just that. If they later feel I am not or they never really thought I was, then that's fine too.

You do you, boo. I'm not here to try and change you.

EPILOGUE

I was shy and quiet and wasn't one to disobey. I would watch the older kids get in trouble and face the blunt edge of their consequences. As a result, I learned, early on, what not to do. I followed the rules, I didn't want to be or feel at fault, and to this day, I hate being the one who did something wrong—not that I can't accept the fault; I just internally beat myself up for any perceived mistakes. I'm really hard on myself.

Ironically enough, I had a period in my life where I flew to the beat of my own drum; where others' opinions didn't matter when they were negative. I was extremely confident and felt very much like someone who people were just drawn towards. I had many boyfriends in high school (not all at once, mind you), but I typically wasn't single for long. I wish I had appreciated the attention more at that time because now, it feels merely impossible to grasp a man's attention for very long. It's like they have ADD, but really, I feel it's just that they're "scared of a relationship with the chick in the wheelchair."

Maybe I still have some work to do to get to a place where I feel as confident as I did as a teenager, but there were also so few responsibilities at that age, to where having a carefree perspective was all I knew.

I've experienced more struggles so far than some ever do—or at least don't have to until they're much older. It isn't common to be faced with a debilitating disease at the ripe age of twenty-one. I have had to relearn so many life tasks. No wonder I am constantly stressed and my body feels hard as a rock from all the tension. I am always, always, always having to be on full alert, for every movement I make. There is the chance I could fall and have to cancel plans. There's the possibility I'm too tired and can't drive to my friend's. And I have a child, so canceling or postponing plans can't always happen. I really do my exercises, workouts, diets, sleep patterns, and activities solely for my kid. Being there and being *present* are two different things and it is important to me to be a hands-on and reliable mom.

Today, I took my son to the doctor and as we were leaving, I took the paperwork the doc handed to me and put it on my lap to start wheeling to the exit as the doc said, "Give those papers to Eli. He can carry them." I did hand them to Eli to carry, but in all honesty, I probably wouldn't have even thought to give them to him to hold if the doctor hadn't said something. I think it's because I already have to ask him to do things an average child doesn't have to do, and so to make up for that, I do absolutely all of what I am capable. He pushed me into the building, so I felt I should at least carry the papers. I catch myself questioning: *What's too much, too little, too hard, too easy for Eli?* I need to be better at always doing what works for me and Eli, rather than taking others' comments to any great length.

One thing I really wish was easier for me, and for both Eli's and my life, is disability support. I mean, why are disability checks in such a small amount that make it extremely difficult to live comfortably? It's like, "Hey if you wanna live above the poverty line, you've gotta put forth the same work ethic as this other thirty-year-old who can walk." Like what the hell?! I hear comments that handicapped individuals are mouthy and want the world to bend over for them. *Umm no.* Maybe if we're not treated like dirt and get enough money to live better than a peasant, we wouldn't have to stress about falling every time we go to pee. Why can't organizations that want to help be more helpful?

As thankful as I am for the vocational rehab and fundraisers and scholarships that support me, I've probably lost a lot of sleep, gained so much stress, and spent and drained so much energy into phone calls, applications, and interviews… It always feels like I'm this convict trying so hard for someone to believe me and to take me seriously. I wonder if anyone else who's disabled feels this way. Like, why aren't they knocking on my door saying, "I'm here to help, no need to stress so much"?

I think that's what I'm yearning for. Someone to take the reigns in what should be the simplicities of life. When dealing with pain that's pretty constant, you can get really emotional and things hit harder. Everyday life hits harder. I have to be patient, soooo patient, and while I feel this has made me a kinder, more generous, more loving and *much* stronger person, I often experience doubt about it all.

Did I *want* to have to become this person, so kind and generous and patient? No… honestly, I just wanted to have fun forever, have a family, and laugh a lot. But did *life* need for me to become this person? I think it did. I like to think that I am making the world a better place through how I hold what has been handed to me to carry. I like to think there's a method to this madness, and, honestly, whether there is a purpose to it all or not, I'm going to move forward as though there is, because of how it facilitates faith. And hope. How it allows me to persevere each new symptom, each daily physical challenge.

Hope has become my shield, and love the sword I wield, in fighting this uphill battle with Friedreich's Ataxia. As far as I'm concerned, FA will never fucking win.

AFTERWORD

Hello, Reader. If you're like me, you've just finished reading Erin's incredible memoir and are turning the pages hoping for more. I'm Hayley, one of Erin's cousins from her large extended family. It's a pleasure to meet you, and an honor to be a part of this.

Erin and I are two years apart and lived just minutes away from each other, growing up friends as equally as cousins. Getting to spend time with her always has and still is what I look forward to most about all of the birthday, holiday, and "just because" get-togethers. When we were kids, we were always on the move—whether jumping on the trampoline, playing Sharks-n-Minnows at the pool, or trying to pull an all-nighter during sleepovers. I used to get so excited when my mom said our plans for the day were "running to Erin's," then just as quickly disappointed to learn she actually had said "running errands." Not much changed, the older we got——I always admired my cool, older, hottie of a cousin and have her to thank (or maybe blame) for wanting to wear makeup and shave my legs before others my age were doing so.

Erin is the type of person who lights up a room whenever she enters. Whether you're meeting her for the first time or you're a close friend, she listens, asks questions, and recalls things from previous conversations or encounters. She is the type of person that is inclusive of everyone at the table; so effortless to connect and laugh with, you can't help but walk away feeling genuinely warm and fulfilled. If, while reading, you were ever thinking, *Is she really this optimistic of a person?* Or, *How can she maintain the turning-lemons-into-lemonade mentality with everything she's endured?* Well, as a self-appointed character witness, I'm here to affirm she *is* all of that... and so much more.

I'll never forget the moment Erin announced her pregnancy. It was Thanksgiving and the entire family stood in a circle around the feast, having just finished up a prayer, and were ready to throw some blows to be the first in line to eat. Erin said that she had an announcement to make, then shared that she was expecting. I recall there being several seconds of silence after she spoke, although those seconds must've felt like a deafening eternity to her, before my mom jumped across the circle with a big "Congratulations!!" and a hug, opening the floodgates for excitement and collective dreaming out loud about the serendipitous future.

As excited as we were for the big news, I know we all shared concerns about how pregnancy would impact Erin's FA progression and the health of the baby. I'd like to think it was in that moment where we all recognized that shared vulnerability, and rallied around this sweet baby that was about to make Erin's dreams come true by making her a mother.

Eli is an incredibly bright boy, inheriting many of the traits we cherish in Erin. Whether it's dinosaurs, US presidents, or sharks, he's always soaking up everything he can about an interesting topic until he's mastered it and is ready for the next one. Brains aside, he possesses so many qualities that aren't learned in a textbook—he's kind, well-mannered, inclusive, and attentive—all simply because he witnesses and emulates those intangibles in his daily life. Eli is yet another gift Erin has given this world.

I, too, hope you've found what you were looking for when you picked up this book, or at a minimum, I hope as you turn the final page, you feel genuinely warm and fulfilled just as you would walking away from any interaction with Erin.

—Hayley Davis

Acknowledgements

First and foremost, my mom deserves the biggest acknowledgment for tons of support and feedback throughout my writing journey. My mom is the person who reads all my rough drafts so I can hear the words I've written out loud. Her opinion always means the most and I've gotten this far with her guidance. My mom is one of my favorite humans and has a heart of gold.

My other favorite human is my son, Eli. Being his mom gave me so much power—the power to embark on writing a story for the world to read. Having FA and Eli are the two main reasons why this story came to fruition.

To my mom and dad, as a whole, for giving me a place to live and revamping your home with all the handicap necessities. And the biggest thank you of all for lending a helping hand to help raise my son, your grandson. Your selflessness never goes unnoticed.

To my cousin Elise and her family, for giving trips and vacations for Eli and me and always accommodating my needs. We've built some wonderful memories.

Alyssa, Joe, Kelly, Mark and Shaun: Thank you for organizing and putting forth all the effort in making a fundraiser for me to continue travels for research trials, what a wonderful hit and success. An unforgettable day!

To the Pieper and Wild families, thank you for the 'beating FA on the fairway' golf tournament fundraiser. The funds helped me to continue research trials and tune up my much-needed modifications and accommodations at home.

I thank my big family and friends for always pushing me with kind and motivational words to write a book. It is because of your encouraging me to write more, because you thought my blog posts were "beautifully" written, that I was able to do this.

And a big thank you to all my 'FAns' cheering me on in any way; this has brought me to such a happier place!

My cousin Hayley, thank you for helping me get some words on paper. Listening to me talk about certain chapters and being my fingers to type.

And thank you to every one of you who has ever assisted someone who needs it. Thank you to each of you who choose to not judge the book by the cover, and really get to know someone, no matter the conditions of their life. I thank you.

ABOUT THE AUTHOR

Erin Pieper is a single mom who advocates for finding a treatment for Friedreich's Ataxia (FA), a rare disease she is faced with. She volunteers as an Ambassador for FARA (Friedreich's Ataxia Research Alliance) on their blogging team. She writes about individuals who are introducing themselves to the FA community, as well as on different fundraising events and their outcomes.

Erin has participated in many fundraising events, near and far, and has taken part in more than five research drug trials at the University of South Florida, in hopes of finding a treatment for FA. She is the designer of FAn, a t-shirt campaign that advocates that the purchaser and /or wearer is a fan of spreading awareness and support for those diagnosed with FA. Get yours to show support here: https://www.bonfire.com/store/fan/

She spends a lot of her time overcoming the struggles of FA, in order to be as involved of a mom as possible, and make the world a kinder place.

Erin would love for you to comment about this book on your favorite social media platform, connect via call or text, or come on over to her place for a chat!

Visit her blog: www.mywobblyworld.com
(Or at least be friends on the socials so we can stalk each other.)
Facebook: Erin Pieper
Instagram: @peepr

ABOUT THE PUBLISHER

S M O K E B L O O D

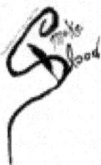

Publishing for the New Paradigm

SMOKEBLOOD serves as a conscious collective supporting
creators through sustainability, transparency and collaboration.
"The whole thing is a weaving of smoke." —Alan Watts

If you'd like to publish your own book, or for bulk discounts,
please contact the publisher directly:

IG: @_smokeblood
connect@smokebloodpublishing.com
www.smokeblood.com